OBSTETRIC
ANESTHESIA

Quick References & Practical Guides

OBSTETRIC ANESTHESIA
Quick References & Practical Guides

Philip E. Hess, MD

*Executive Vice Chair, Department of Anesthesia, Critical Care and Pain Medicine,
Beth Israel Deaconess Medical Center, Associate Professor in Anaesthesia,
Associate Professor of Obstetrics, Gynecology, and Reproductive Biology,
Harvard Medical School, Boston, Massachusetts*

Yunping Li, MD

*Director, Obstetric Anesthesia, Department of Anesthesia, Critical Care and Pain Medicine,
Beth Israel Deaconess Medical Center, Associate Professor in Anaesthesia,
Assistant Professor of Obstetrics, Gynecology, and Reproductive Biology,
Harvard Medical School, Boston, Massachusetts*

John J. Kowalczyk, MD

*Section Head of Anesthesia for Gynecology Surgery, Department of Anesthesia,
Critical Care and Pain Medicine, Beth Israel Deaconess Medical Center, Instructor in Anaesthesia,
Harvard Medical School, Boston, Massachusetts*

Justin K. Stiles, MD

*Department of Anesthesia, Critical Care and Pain Medicine, Beth Israel Deaconess Medical Center,
Instructor in Anaesthesia, Harvard Medical School, Boston, Massachusetts*

New York   Chicago   San Francisco   Athens   London   Madrid   Mexico City
New Delhi   Milan   Singapore   Sydney   Toronto

Obstetric Anesthesia: Quick References & Practical Guides

1 2 3 4 5 6 7 DSS 26 25 24 23

ISBN 978-1-264-67146-5

MHID 1-264-67146-6

This book was set in Minion Pro by MPS Limited.
The editors were Timothy Y. Hiscock and Kim J. Davis.
The production supervisor was Richard Ruzycka.
Project management was provided by Poonam Bisht of MPS Limited.
The cover design was W2 Design.

This book is printed on acid-free paper.

Library of Congress Cataloging-in-Publication Data

Names: Hess, Philip E., contributor, editor. | Li, Yunping, contributor,
  editor. | Kowalczyk, John J., contributor, editor. | Stiles, Justin K.,
  contributor, editor.
Title: Obstetric anesthesia : quick references & practical guides / [edited
  by] Philip E. Hess, Yunping Li, John J. Kowalczyk, Justin K. Stiles.
Other titles: Obstetric anesthesia (Hess)
Description: New York : McGraw Hill, [2023] | Includes bibliographical
  references and index. | Summary: "This textbook features a succinct,
  evidence-based review tied with practical and clinical protocols for
  each important topic in the anesthetic care of the pregnant woman"—
  Provided by publisher.
Identifiers: LCCN 2022044899 (print) | LCCN 2022044900 (ebook) |
  ISBN 9781264671465 (paperback ; alk. paper) | ISBN 9781264671472 (ebook)
Subjects: MESH: Anesthesia, Obstetrical—methods | Pregnancy Complications
  | Anesthetics | Obstetric Labor Complications | Handbook
Classification: LCC RG732 (print) | LCC RG732 (ebook) | NLM WO 231 |
  DDC 617.9/682—dc23/eng/20221230
LC record available at https://lccn.loc.gov/2022044899
LC ebook record available at https://lccn.loc.gov/2022044900

This book is dedicated to my wife, Marika, who sticks by me no matter how stupid I am, my son, Steven, and to the hundreds of anesthesiologists, obstetricians, nurses, and scrub techs who have helped make our team better. And to Yunping Li for pushing us to publish!

Philip E. Hess

This book is dedicated to the memory of my mother Zhanmei Zhang and to my father Yifei Li for their encouragement; to my husband, Weixing, who supports me daily; to my son, Kevin, who has honored me by pursuing a career as a physician.

Yunping Li

To all those who have taken the time to listen and provide me their wisdom throughout my career. And to my wife, Revital, for her support and ability to remind me that the imperfect can be amazing.

John J. Kowalczyk

To my wife, Kristen and my amazing twin daughters, Sophie and Lucy.

Justin K. Stiles

Contents

Contributors

Vimal K. Akhouri, MD
Department of Anesthesia, Critical Care and Pain Medicine
Beth Israel Deaconess Medical Center
Instructor in Anaesthesia, Harvard Medical School
Boston, Massachusetts

Amnon A. Berger, MD, PhD
Department of Anesthesia, Critical Care and Pain Medicine
Beth Israel Deaconess Medical Center
Boston, Massachusetts

Maria C. Borrelli, DO
Director, Medical Student Education
Department of Anesthesia, Critical Care and Pain Medicine
Beth Israel Deaconess Medical Center
Instructor in Anaesthesia
Harvard Medical School
Boston, Massachusetts

Erin J. Ciampa, MD, PhD
Department of Anesthesia, Critical Care and Pain Medicine
Beth Israel Deaconess Medical Center
Assistant Professor in Anaesthesia
Harvard Medical School
Boston, Massachusetts

Merry I. Colella, MD
Director, Residency Education in Obstetric Anesthesia
Department of Anesthesia, Critical Care and Pain Medicine
Beth Israel Deaconess Medical Center
Instructor in Anaesthesia
Harvard Medical School
Boston, Massachusetts

Susan Craft, RN, MS
Beth Israel Deaconess Medical Center
Boston, Massachusetts

Janet C. Guarino, RN, MS
Nursing Director Labor and Delivery
Beth Israel Deaconess Medical Center
Boston, Massachusetts

Josephine M. Hernandez, MD
Vice Chair, Department of Anesthesia, Critical Care and Pain Medicine
Beth Israel Deaconess Medical Center
Assistant Professor in Anaesthesia
Harvard Medical School
Boston, Massachusetts

Philip E. Hess, MD
Executive Vice Chair, Department of Anesthesia, Critical Care and Pain Medicine
Beth Israel Deaconess Medical Center
Associate Professor in Anaesthesia, Associate Professor of Obstetrics, Gynecology, and Reproductive Biology
Harvard Medical School
Boston, Massachusetts

Mohammed Idris, MD
Department of Anesthesia, Critical Care and Pain Medicine
Beth Israel Deaconess Medical Center
Boston, Massachusetts

Colin B. Jackson, MD
Department of Obstetrics and Gynecology
Beth Israel Deaconess Medical Center
Boston, Massachusetts

Galina V. Korsunsky, MD
Department of Anesthesia, Critical Care and Pain Medicine
Beth Israel Deaconess Medical Center
Instructor in Anaesthesia
Harvard Medical School
Boston, Massachusetts

John J. Kowalczyk, MD
Section Head of Anesthesia for Gynecology Surgery
Department of Anesthesia, Critical Care and Pain Medicine
Beth Israel Deaconess Medical Center
Instructor in Anaesthesia
Harvard Medical School
Boston, Massachusetts

Lior Levy, MD
Director, Simulation for Residency Education
Department of Anesthesia, Critical Care and Pain Medicine
Beth Israel Deaconess Medical Center
Instructor in Anaesthesia
Harvard Medical School
Boston, Massachusetts

Yunping Li, MD
Director, Obstetric Anesthesia
Department of Anesthesia, Critical Care and Pain Medicine
Beth Israel Deaconess Medical Center
Associate Professor in Anaesthesia
Assistant Professor of Obstetrics, Gynecology, and
Reproductive Biology
Harvard Medical School
Boston, Massachusetts

Minxian Liang, MD
Department of Anesthesia, Critical Care and Pain Medicine
Beth Israel Deaconess Medical Center
Boston, Massachusetts

Patsy J. McGuire, MD
Department of Anesthesia, Critical Care and Pain
Medicine
Beth Israel Deaconess Medical Center
Instructor in Anaesthesia
Harvard Medical School
Boston, Massachusetts

Anna Moldysz, MD
Department of Anesthesia, Critical Care and Pain Medicine
Beth Israel Deaconess Medical Center
Boston, Massachusetts

Liberty G. Reforma, MD
Division of Maternal-Fetal Medicine
Department of Obstetrics and Gynecology
Beth Israel Deaconess Medical Center
Boston, Massachusetts

Dillon A. Schafer, MD
Department of Anesthesia, Critical Care and Pain Medicine
Beth Israel Deaconess Medical Center
Boston, Massachusetts

Scott A. Shainker, DO, MS
The Annie and Chase Koch Chair in Obstetrics and
Gynecology
Director, New England Center for Placental Disorder
Division of Maternal-Fetal Medicine
Department of Obstetrics and Gynecology
Beth Israel Deaconess Medical Center

Assistant Professor of Obstetrics, Gynecology, and
Reproductive Biology
Harvard Medical School
Boston, Massachusetts

Aidan Sharkey, MD
Department of Anesthesia, Critical Care and Pain Medicine
Beth Israel Deaconess Medical Center
Instructor in Anaesthesia
Harvard Medical School
Boston, Massachusetts

Joan E. Spiegel, MD
Department of Anesthesia, Critical Care and Pain Medicine
Beth Israel Deaconess Medical Center
Assistant Professor in Anaesthesia
Harvard Medical School
Boston, Massachusetts

Justin K. Stiles, MD
Department of Anesthesia, Critical Care and Pain
Medicine
Beth Israel Deaconess Medical Center
Instructor in Anaesthesia
Harvard Medical School
Boston, Massachusetts

Jordan B. Strom, MD, MSc
Department of Cardiology
Associate Director, Echocardiography Laboratory
Director of Echocardiographic Research,
Division of Cardiovascular Medicine
Beth Israel Deaconess Medical Center
Section Head, Cardiovascular Imaging Research, Richard
A. and Susan F. Smith Center for Outcomes Research in
Cardiology
Assistant Professor of Medicine
Harvard Medical School
Boston, Massachusetts

Lindsay K. Sween, MD, MPH
Department of Anesthesia, Critical Care and Pain Medicine
Beth Israel Deaconess Medical Center
Boston, Massachusetts

Sichao Xu, MD
Department of Anesthesia, Critical Care and Pain Medicine
Beth Israel Deaconess Medical Center
Boston, Massachusetts

Liana Zucco, MD, MBBS
Department of Anaesthesia
Guy's and St Thomas' NHS Foundation Trust
London, United Kingdom

Preface

Obstetric Anesthesia: Quick References & Practical Guides is a new book designed for clinicians and for their obstetric anesthesia practices.

Several high-quality textbooks have been published that provide detailed understanding of the current science behind obstetrics and obstetric anesthesia. *Obstetric Anesthesia: Quick References & Practical Guides* complements existing textbooks by assisting learners and clinicians with concise answers and applicable clinical pathways. By condensing most topics into short, evidence-based description and clinically useful tables and charts, a busy clinician can find the answer to a question, learn clinical pearls. This book represents a collection of common and uncommon clinical challenges with up-to-date obstetric anesthesia practices that serve both experienced and novice clinicians.

This book also supports the obstetric anesthesia practice by providing easily adaptable pathways, protocols, and standard operating procedures. Standard work has been a guiding principle in the manufacturing industry for over a century. As stated by a founding father of Toyota's manufacturing, Taiichi Ohno, "Without standards, there can be no improvement." Only recently has medicine begun to explore the idea of standardization, not just of clinical work but also the working environment. This crucial evolution in medicine will lead to better outcomes for patients, providers, and trainees.

The training of anesthesia providers has historically been performed using an apprenticeship model. We all learned from our teachers, who learned from theirs, and so forth. There was little uniformity in training. Even large training programs have clinicians with differing knowledge and practice styles. At times this can be confusing, as the clinician of the day may do things that are the opposite of the clinician from the day before. Gradually, medical education has evolved from this apprenticeship model to evidence-based medicine, whereby clinicians address problems in a similar fashion.

Over 20 years ago, the obstetric anesthesia service at Beth Israel Deaconess Medical Center began the evolution from an individual clinician practice to a group practice where each of us practices similarly. To do this, we implemented practice protocols and standard operating procedures based on the best scientific evidence. At the same time, we started an intense quality improvement program to understand where our failures were and how they could be improved. The lessons we learned are enmeshed in this book. While our information will need to be adapted to local environments, we believe that the value of a shared model of clinical practice is extremely rewarding and essential for patient care.

We sincerely hope that by providing our clinical tips, guidelines, and protocols, we can further the clinical improvement of obstetric anesthesia.

Philip E. Hess, MD
Yunping Li, MD
John J. Kowalczyk, MD
Justin K. Stiles, MD

Acknowledgments

The editors gratefully acknowledge contributing authors; they are outstanding physicians who dedicate themselves for care of pregnant women. Their expertise, wisdom, and hard work have made this book possible.

We are indebted to Daniel Talmor, MD for his constructive advice and generous support, and to Heather Derocher for her assistance in publishing.

We acknowledge the expertise, encouragement, and support provided by the professional production team at McGraw Hill.

PART I
GENERAL INFORMATION

1

Common Medications

Yunping Li, MD

Azithromycin	• 500 mg, diluted in 20 mL of normal saline (NS)/lactated Ringers, infusion slowly over 1 hour. • 4 mg of Ondansetron intravenously (IV) before infusion due to significant nausea and vomiting. • Indications: intrapartum cesarean section, spontaneous rupture of membrane. Reference: *N Engl J Med.* 2016;375:1231-1241.
Bicitra	• Generic name: sodium citrate/citric acid; 30 mL per container. • Per os (PO), before epidural placement and before cesarean delivery.
Chloroprocaine	• 3% chloroprocaine, preservative free (PF). • Alkalization: In a 30-mL syringe, add 2 mL of 8.4% bicarbonate to 20 mL of chloroprocaine. • Use for emergent cesarean delivery or for forceps delivery. • **STAT Cesarean Kit:** Prepackage in obstetric anesthesia office: (1) 3% chloroprocaine; (1) 8.4% bicarbonate; (1) 30-mL syringe; (1) blunt needle. Replace it after use.

Dexmedetomidine	• Dilute 200 µg in 20 mL of NS, final concentration 10 µg/mL.
	• Indications:
	  ○ Severe shivering after delivery: 10 µg IV, may repeat up to 30 µg.
	  ○ Severe pruritus associated with epidural fentanyl, see Chapter 6.
	Reference: *Int J Obstet Anesth.* 2021;45:49-55.

Ephedrine	• Premixed by pharmacy, 5 mg/mL. • Historically, ephedrine was used as the "Gold standard" for spinal hypotension. • Higher placental transfer than phenylephrine; it can cause clinically insignificant fetal acidosis. • Since late 1990s, used as a second-line medicine for maternal hypotension. References: *Am J Obstet Gynecol.* 1968;102:911. *Anesthesiology.* 2009;111:506-512.

Epinephrine	• Add 250 μg to 150 mL premixed bupivacaine/fentanyl epidural solution; final concentration will be 1.67 μg/mL.
	• Add 5 μg/mL of epinephrine into 2% lidocaine for cesarean delivery.
	• Mechanisms: alpha-2 synergic effect, alpha-1 vasoconstriction to prolong the duration of anesthesia and decrease systemic absorption. Reference: *J Anesth Perioper Med.* 2019;6:1-7.

Lidocaine	• 2% lidocaine, PF.
	• Alkalization of lidocaine: in a 30-mL syringe, add 2 mL of 8.4% bicarbonate to 20 mL of lidocaine.
	• For cesarean delivery, add 5 μg/mL of epinephrine.

Magnesium	• 2 g/h infusion as maintenance dose.
	• For preeclampsia, continue magnesium for entire cesarean delivery.
	• For fetal neuroprotection, discontinue magnesium after delivery. Reference: The Magpie Trial. *Lancet.* 2002;359:1877-1890.

| Morphine | • 0.5 mL/mL, PF, pre-made by pharmacy, stored at 4°C. |
| | • Indications:
  ○ Cesarean delivery—spinal 250 μg, epidural 3 mg.
  ○ Labor CSE for dysfunctional labor—spinal 100 μg.
  ○ After third degree vaginal laceration repair—epidural 2 mg.
Refer to Chapters 2, 41, and 42 for details. |

Nitroglycerin	• 400 μg/mL, light sensitive. Kept in Omnicell in the operating room. Dilute to 100 μg/mL.
	• Dose: 100 μg IV, may repeat, titrate to effect.
	• Indications: cervico-uterine relaxation, inverted uterus, difficult extraction at cesarean delivery. Reference: *Am J Obstet Gynecol.* 1998;179:813.

Phenylephrine	• Pre-made by pharmacy, 100 μg/mL.
	• Indications: first-line medication for maternal hypotension.
	• Phenylephrine use is associated with a decrease in maternal cardiac output, but the clinical significance is not clear.
	• Infusion at 0.5 to 0.7 μg/kg/min or bolus 100 μg, titrate to effect. Reference: *Anesth Analg.* 2012;114:377.

| Terbutaline | • 1 mg/mL, use 0.25 mg, subcutaneously, administrated by the nurse. |
| | • Indications:
  ○ Tachysystole contraction with associated fetal heart rate changes.
  ○ Before external cephalic version at obstetrician's discretion.
ACOG Practice Bulletin No. 106. |

Tranexamic Acid	• Tranexamic acid (TXA) 1 g, diluted in 20 mL of NS, infuse over 10 min. • Treatment of postpartum hemorrhage (PPH) after vaginal or cesarean delivery. • Prophylaxis in high risk of PPH (e.g., women with hypertensive disorder and asthma). • Discourage use of TXA for prophylaxis in low-risk women (no proven benefit). • Exclusion: History of deep vein thrombosis/pulmonary embolism/myocardial infarction/cerebrovascular accident, acquired color blindness. • Decreased dose (5 mg/kg) for renal failure. Refer to Chapter 3 for details. References: *N Engl J Med.* 2018;379:731-742. 　　　　　　*Lancet.* 2017;389:2105-2116.
Uterotonics	• Including oxytocin, methylergonovine (methergine), carboprost (hemabate), misoprostol (Cytotec), and calcium chloride. Refer to Chapter 5 for details.

2

Dosage Cookbook

Philip E. Hess, MD

Dosage Cookbook

FOR LABOR	FOR CESAREAN
Spinal Analgesia Bupivacaine 2 mg Fentanyl 12.5 µg *Premixed by pharmacy, stored at 4°C in the Omnicell* **MIX** 0.8 mL of Bupivacaine (0.25%) with 0.25 mL of Fentanyl (50 µg/mL)	**Spinal Anesthesia** Bupivacaine 11.25 mg Fentanyl 25 µg Morphine, PF 150-250 µg **MIX** 1.5 mL of Bupivacaine (0.75%, hyperbaric) 0.5 mL of Fentanyl (50 µg/mL) 0.3-0.5 mL of PF Morphine (0.5 mg/mL)
Labor Epidural Analgesia 0.04% Bupivacaine 1.67 µg/mL Fentanyl 1.67 µg/mL Epinephrine (may add 0.25 mL of 1:1000 epinephrine) *Premixed by pharmacy, stored at 4°C in the Omnicell* **TOP-UP:** 0.0625% Bupivacaine 10-15 mL OR 0.125% Bupivacaine 5-10 mL Add 50-100 µg of Fentanyl for synergy	**Epidural Anesthesia** **MIX** Lidocaine 2% 20 mL Sodium bicarbonate 8.4% 2 mL Epinephrine 1:1000 0.1 mL Inject divided doses, 3-5 mL at a time. Bolus 50 µg/mL Fentanyl 2 mL between the doses After delivery: give PF Morphine 3 mg. Lidocaine may be replaced with 3% Chloroprocaine or 0.5% Bupivacaine (with caution)

Bicarbonation
 	
                 Drug   Bicarbonate
2% Lidocaine   20 mL   2 mL
3% Chloroprocaine 20 mL   2 mL
0.5% Bupivacaine 10 mL   0.1 mL
(will precipitate with Bupivacaine)
	Uterotonics
	
	Oxytocin: 20 IU in 1 L of LR
	     Beware hypotension
	Methylergonovine: 0.2 mg IM **not** IV
	     Beware hypertension
	Carboprost: 250 µg IM **not** IV
	     Beware bronchospasm
	Misoprostol: 1 mg PR
	     Beware fever and rigor

IM, intramuscular; IV, intravenous; LR, lactated Ringers; PF, preservative free; PR, per rectum.

3

Tranexamic Acid

Philip E. Hess, MD

BACKGROUND

Obstetric hemorrhage is the leading cause of maternal mortality worldwide. Despite active management during the third stage of labor, postpartum hemorrhage (PPH) remains a problem and is increasing in the United States, primarily due to the increasing incidence of atony.[1] Tranexamic acid (TXA) is a lysine analogue and works by binding to plasminogen, thereby inhibiting fibrinolysis. TXA has been used for years in the management and prevention of hemorrhage in the surgical setting, including cardiac, orthopedic, and trauma surgery.[2,3]

Prior studies have established the safety and efficacy of using TXA in the treatment of PPH. More recently, a large, international, multicenter, randomized control trial (The WOMAN trial) demonstrated a significant reduction in PPH and death due to bleeding when TXA was used early in the treatment of PPH.[4] Although there is less data, several studies have demonstrated its efficacy in preventing PPH in patients at both average or increased risk when given immediately after delivery in cesarean deliveries.[5-7] Conversely, large randomized studies have shown modest to no benefit of prophylactic TXA to prevent PPH in healthy parturients undergoing vaginal delivery compared to placebo.[8-10] Despite concerns for potentially increasing thromboembolic events, no study to date has indicated any increased risk in gravid patients receiving TXA. Given this data, our goals are outlined below.

GOALS

- To reduce the severity of PPH once a patient has been identified as having excessive bleeding (estimated blood loss >500 mL in vaginal delivery or >1000 mL in vaginal delivery or cesarean delivery).
- To reduce the incidence of PPH in patients at high-risk for hemorrhage due to known risk factors.

CLINICAL PRACTICE

- Therapeutic use: Consider use when patient has been identified as having a hemorrhage. Team agreement prior to administration.
- Prophylactic use: Consider prophylactic use in cesarean or vaginal delivery with patients at increased risk for hemorrhage (see criteria below), especially in circumstances where uterotonics may be contraindicated. Discuss possible use at briefing or at team meeting.

METHOD OF ADMINISTRATION

Dosage: 1 g given intravenously over 10 minutes. Possible methods of administration include 1 g diluted into 10 ml of normal saline or 1 g diluted into 100 ml of normal saline.

Timing: Administer when hemorrhage has been identified. In high-risk patients where prophylactic administration has been agreed upon, initiate **immediately** after delivery of baby in either vaginal or cesarean delivery. Consider redosing 1 g after 30 minutes of continuing hemorrhage. Consider infusion (5 mg/kg/h) if prolonged bleeding period is expected.

SIDE EFFECTS

Minor: nausea, vomiting, gastrointestinal upset, headaches, dizziness, hypotension, color blindness

Major: thromboembolic complications, e.g., pulmonary embolism (PE), deep vein thrombosis (DVT), myocardial infarction, seizure, anaphylaxis

Caution: mistakenly administration of TXA into epidural or subarachnoid space can cause intractable seizure; deaths had been reported.

AT INCREASED RISK FOR HEMORRHAGE

- Abnormal placentation (previa, placenta accreta spectrum)
- Polyhydramnios
- History of prior PPH
- Multiple gestations
- Grand multiparity
- Chorioamnionitis
- Fetal macrosomia (fetal weight >5000 g)
- Morbid obesity (BMI >40 kg/m^2)
- Known coagulopathy
- Retained placenta
- Suspected placental abruption
- Prolonged induction

CONTRAINDICATIONS

- History of thromboembolic disease (DVT, PE, or cerebral vascular accident)
- History of ischemic heart disease
- Known disorder of hypercoagulability (e.g., Factor V Leiden)
- Prior reaction to TXA

RELATIVE CONTRAINDICATIONS

- Oliguria

References

1. Kramer S, Berg C, Abehmaim H, et al. Incidence, risk factors and temporal trends in severe postpartum hemorrhage. *Am J Obstet Gynecol*. 2013;209(5):449.e1-449e.7.
2. Cheriyan T, Maier SP 2nd, Bianco K, et al. Efficacy of tranexamic acid on surgical bleeding in spine surgery: a meta-analysis. *Spine J*. 2015;15(4):752-761.

3. CRASH-2 Trial Collaborators, Shakur H, Roberts I, Bautista R, et al. Effects of tranexamic acid on death, vascular occlusive events, and blood transfusion in trauma patients with significant hemorrhage (CRASH 2): a randomized placebo-controlled trial. *Lancet*. 2010;376:23-32.

4. WOMAN Trial Collaborators. Effect of early tranexamic acid administration on mortality, hysterectomy, and other morbidities in women with postpartum haemorrhage (WOMAN): an international, randomized, double-blind, placebo-controlled trial. *Lancet*. 2017;389:2105-2116.

5. Sujata N, Tobin R, Kaur R, et al. Randomized controlled trial of tranexamic acid among parturients at increased risk for postpartum hemorrhage undergoing cesarean delivery. *Int J Gynaecol Obstet*. 2016;133:312-315.

6. Bellos I, Pergialiotis V. Tranexamic acid for the prevention of postpartum hemorrhage in women undergoing cesarean delivery: an updated meta-analysis. *J Matern Fetal Neonatal Med*. 2020;33(19):3368-3376.

7. Sentilhes L, Sénat MV, Le Lous M, et al. Tranexamic acid for the prevention of blood loss after cesarean delivery. *N Engl J Med*. 2021;384(17):1623-1634.

8. Saccone G, Della Corte L, D'Alessandro P, et al. Prophylactic use of tranexamic acid after vaginal delivery reduces the risk of primary postpartum hemorrhage. *J Matern Fetal Neonatal Med*. 2020;33(19):3368-3376.

9. Gungorduk K, Asicioglu O, Yildirim G, et al. Can intravenous injection of tranexamic acid be used in routine practice with active management of the third stage of labor in vaginal delivery? A randomized controlled study. *Am J Perinatol*. 2013;30(5):407-413.

10. Sentilhes L, Winer N, Azria E, et al. Tranexamic acid for the prevention of blood loss after vaginal delivery. *N Engl J Med*. 2018;379(8):731-742.

4

Oxytocin

Yunping Li, MD

MECHANISM

Oxytocin binds to a G-protein–coupled receptor. Activation triggers elevation of intracellular calcium that stimulates uterine smooth muscle contraction. Its function is regulated by:

- Changes in receptor expression
- Receptor internalization leading to oxytocin desensitization
- Local changes in oxytocin concentration

PRECAUTIONS

The effects of oxytocin on vascular smooth muscles depend on types of vasculatures and vascular basal tones. While oxytocin induces uterine contractions, higher concentration of oxytocin relaxes the high-resistance vasculatures of skeleton muscles, liver, kidney, and spleen.[1] Rapid injection of a large dose of oxytocin in severe hypovolemic patients with postpartum hemorrhage may result in worsening hypotension, myocardial ischemia, circulatory collapse, and even maternal death.[2]

Large total oxytocin doses should be avoided to minimize the antidiuretic effect. The patient on high dose of oxytocin for induction of labor for a prolong period could be at increased risk to develop severe hyponatremia or seizure.

DOSAGE AND ADMINISTRATION[3]

Standardized oxytocin protocols have been shown to reduce the incidence of postpartum hemorrhage.[4] Oxytocin should be given as a small initial dose after delivery, followed by a controlled infusion. Oxytocin dose requirements are higher for intrapartum cesarean deliveries.[5] FDA mandates to use infusion pump for oxytocin administration (Fig. 4-1).

A second-line medication (ergot or prostaglandins) should be considered **EARLY** if oxytocin fails to produce good uterine tone.

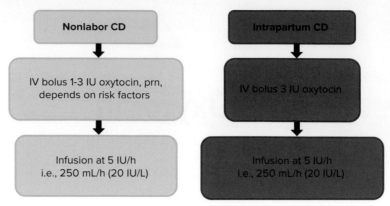

FIGURE 4-1 • Administration of oxytocin for cesarean delivery.

References

1. Altura BM, Altura BT. Actions of vasopressin, oxytocin, and synthetic analogs on vascular smooth muscle. *Fed Proc*. 1984;43(1):80-86.

2. Bolton TJ, Randall K, Yentis SM. Effect of the confidential enquiries into maternal deaths on the use of Syntocinon at caesarean section in the UK. *Anaesthesia*. 2003;58(3):277-279.

3. Heesen M, Carvalho B, Carvalho JCA, et al. International consensus statement on the use of uterotonic agents during caesarean section. *Anaesthesia*. 2019;74:1305-1319.

4. Doyle JL, Kenny TH, Gothard MD, et al. A standardized oxytocin administration protocol after delivery to reduce the treatment of postpartum hemorrhage. *Jt Comm J Qual Patient Safety*. 2019;45:131-143.

5. Lavoie A, McCarthy RJ, Wong CA. The ED90 of prophylactic oxytocin after delivery of the placenta during Cesarean delivery in laboring compared with nonlaboring women: an up-down sequential allocation dose-response study. *Anesth Analg*. 2015;121:159-164.

5

Uterotonics

Dillon Schafer, MD
Yunping Li, MD

Postpartum hemorrhage (PPH) is a leading cause of maternal mortality, accounting for about 35% of all maternal deaths globally.[1] Uterine atony remains the single most common cause of PPH, responsible for nearly 80% of total cases.[2] Strategy and choice of administrating uterotonic agents are summarized in Table 5-1.

TABLE 5-1 • Strategies of Administrating Uterotonics		
WHO recommends use of an effective uterotonic for prevention of PPH for **all** births	The patients with placenta previa may have PPH despite good uterine tone	If the first-line uterotonics is not efficient, choose the second-line medication immediately

OXYTOCIN (PITOCIN)—FIRST LINE

Mechanism	Activation of oxytocin receptors in the myometrium. Prolong exposure to oxytocin during labor can lead to receptor desensitization and increase the risk of PPH.[3]
Side effects	When it is given in large intravenous (IV) doses, oxytocin can cause hypotension, tachycardia, and nausea. Oxytocin is structurally similar to antidiuretic hormone; extended use of oxytocin may cause water retention, hyponatremia, and seizures (Chapter 4, "Oxytocin").
How to give	Bolus: For PPH high-risk patients, 3 units IV before infusion. Infusion: 20 units in 1 L of Lactated Ringers, infuse at 250 mL/h (5 IU/h) or 375 mL/h (7.5 IU/h) Intramuscular: 10 units intramuscularly (IM) if no IV catheter.

CARBETOCIN (NOT AVAILABLE IN THE UNITED STATES)—FIRST LINE WHERE ITS COST IS COMPARABLE

Mechanism	Analogue of oxytocin with longer half-life, but more expensive. It is heat stable, suitable for resource-poor countries. Efficacy of carbetocin is noninferior to oxytocin for the prevention of PPH.[4]
Side effects	Hypotension, nausea and vomiting, headache, abdominal pain.
How to give	100 μg IV or IM.

MISOPROSTOL (CYTOTEC)—FIRST LINE IF OXYTOCIN IS UNAVAILABLE

Mechanism	Synthetic analogue of PGE_1. Stimulates uterine smooth muscle contractions. Less potent than carboprost and methylergonovine.
Side effects	Rigors, transient fever, headache, diarrhea, abdominal pain.
How to give	800-1000 µg per rectum; or 400 or 600 µg by mouth, or 800 µg sublingual. Single dose. Stored at room temperature. World Health Organization recommends the administration PO by community or lay healthcare workers where skilled health personnel are not available.

METHYLERGONOVINE (METHERGINE)—SECOND LINE

Mechanism	Serotonin receptor agonist in smooth muscle, particularly within the uterus; partial alpha-adrenergic agonist.
Side effects	Avoid in patients with hypertension, preeclampsia, and Raynaud's syndrome. Other side effects include headache and nausea.
How to give	0.2 mg IM, may repeat in 2-4 hours.

CARBOPROST (HEMABATE)—SECOND LINE

Mechanism	15-methyl $PGF2_{alpha}$, stimulates uterine smooth muscle tonic contractions.
Side effects	May cause bronchospasm, nausea, diarrhea, and hypertension. Avoid in patients with asthma. Relative contraindication for hypertension, active pulmonary or cardiac diseases.
How to give	250 µg IM, may repeat in every 15 minutes, maximum eight doses.

CALCIUM CHLORIDE—ADJUNCTIVE

Mechanism	The second messenger for smooth muscle contraction, including uterus. Magnesium antagonist. May consider it for the patient who is on magnesium with uterine atony.
Side effects	Transient hypertension, bradycardia, arrhythmia.
How to give	1 g IV over 10 minutes.

References

1. Vogel JP, Williams M, Gallos I, et al. WHO recommendations on uterotonics for postpartum haemorrhage prevention: what works, and which one? *BMJ Global Health*. 2019;4:e001466.
2. Bateman BT, Berman MF, Riley LE, Leffert LR. The epidemiology of postpartum hemorrhage in a large, nationwide sample of deliveries. *Anesth Analg*. 2010;110:1368-1373.
3. Arrowsmith S, Wray S. Oxytocin: its mechanism of action and receptor signaling in the myometrium. *J Neuroendocrinol*. 2014;26(6):356-369.
4. Widmer M, Piaggio G, Nguyen TMH, et al. Heat-stable carbetocin versus oxytocin to prevent hemorrhage after vaginal birth. *N Engl J Med*. 2018;379:743-752.

6

Dexmedetomidine

Yunping Li, MD

BACKGROUND

Morphine, fentanyl, sufentanil, and epinephrine have been widely and safely used as adjuvants for labor analgesia and for cesarean delivery anesthesia. An introduction of alpha$_2$-adrenergic agonist dexmedetomidine (DEX) in obstetric anesthesia could provide the unique analgesic benefit without side effects of opioids such as pruritus, urinary retention, hyperalgesia, and respiratory depression. The addition of DEX to neuraxial local anesthetics produces a significant prolongation in the duration of sensory and motor blockage and reduction in post cesarean opioid requirement.[1] Various animal studies have been conducted using intrathecal DEX at a dose range of 2.5 to 100 µg without any neurotoxicity, similarly, without any postoperative neurological deficit in human studies.

CONTROVERSY ON NEURAXIAL DEXMEDETOMIDINE

Approval by the U.S. Food and Drug Administration (FDA) in 1999, DEX is indicated for sedation of ventilated patients in an intensive care setting and sedation for non-intubated patients prior to and/or during surgical procedures.[2]

FDA defines DEX as pregnancy category C medication and suggests that it should be used during pregnancy ONLY if the potential benefits justify the potential risk to the fetus. Of note, although clonidine has been extensively investigated as an adjunct to neuraxial opioids, FDA placed a "black box" for using clonidine in pregnant women due to excessive hypotension and sedation. In the last decade, accumulating clinical data have demonstrated the profound analgesics and safety profile of DEX in obstetric anesthesia. Still, more data are needed to support the use of neuraxial DEX in obstetric anesthesia.

PHARMACOLOGY AND APPLICATIONS[2]

- Highly selective alpha$_2$-adrenergic agonist, the mediator for its analgesic effects.
- Large dose of DEX can cause hypertensive episode due to stimulation of alpha$_{2B}$ receptor.
- Some studies demonstrated neuroprotective effects of intrathecal DEX.[3]
- Octanol: water partition coefficient 2.89, steady volume of distribution of 118 liters.
- Protein binding 94%.
- Maternal/fetal ratio 0.77,[4] high placental retention with negligible placental transfer.
- Preservative free.

- For neuraxial route administration, the onset time for DEX is about 15 minutes; duration of action is about 6 to 8 hours.
- Terminal elimination half-life: 2 hours when given intravenously.
- Can be used for postoperative shivering, replacement of neuraxial opioids to stop pruritus, recurrent breakthrough labor pain, and postsurgical pain.

CLINICAL PRACTICE AND INDICATIONS

- **Intrathecal administration**

Dose	5 or 10 µg in addition to bupivacaine and fentanyl for cesarean delivery
Indications: (1)	Severe pruritus or nausea and vomiting from prior use of neuraxial morphine
(2)	For patients with opioid use disorders as multimodal analgesia (Chapter 16, "Opioid Use Disorders")

- **Epidural administration**

Bolus dose	10-20 µg
Indications: (1)	With functional epidural, consider DEX when patient has recurrent breakthrough pain despite physician-administrated routine bolus (Chapter 42, "Refractory pain during labor epidural analgesia").
(2)	In preparation for cesarean delivery in the patient who had multiple boluses for breakthrough pain during labor. Administrate 10-15 minutes before incision.
(3)	Intolerance to epidural fentanyl/sufentanil for labor analgesia due to severe pruritus. Replace opioids with 0.5 µg/mL DEX for epidural infusion.

- **Intravenous administration**

Dose	10 µg bolus, titrate in with effect, may repeat up to 30 µg in total.
Indication	Severe shivering during cesarean delivery.[5]
	It is not advised to use intravenous infusion for nonobstetric surgery in pregnant women till we have more data to support its use.

SIDE EFFECTS

Clinical application of small doses of DEX in intrathecal and epidural appears safe with minimal side effects.

- Potentiate motor blockage of local anesthetics (LA), if the concentration of LA is high
- Transient hypertension observed primarily with large intravenous loading dose
- Rarely maternal hypotension
- Rarely nausea and vomiting
- Rarely excessive sedation
- Rarely maternal bradycardia
- Dry mouth
- Theoretically fetal bradycardia, with extra low doses in neuraxial administration, fetal bradycardia has not been reported

CONTRAINDICATIONS OR RELATIVE CONTRAINDICATIONS

- Hemodynamically unstable patients
- Bradycardia
- Known allergy to DEX

References

1. Yousef AA, Salem HA, Moustafa MZ. Effect of mini-dose epidural dexmedetomidine in elective cesarean section using combined spinal-epidural anesthesia: a randomized double-blinded controlled study. *J Anaeth.* 2015;29:708-714.

2. https://www.accessdata.fda.gov/drugsatfda_docs/label/2013/021038s021lbl.pdf. Accessed March 2022.

3. Celik F, Gocmez C, Kamasak K, et al. The comparison of neuroprotective effects of intrathecal dexmedetomidine and methylprednisolone in spinal cord injury. *Int J Surg.* 2013;11(5):411-418.

4. Nair AS, Sriprakash K. Dexmedetomidine in pregnancy: Review of literature and possible use. *J Obstet Anaesth Crit Care.* 2013;3:3-6.

5. Sween LK, Xu S, Li C, et al. Low-dose intravenous dexmedetomidine reduces shivering following cesarean delivery: a randomized controlled trial. *Int J Obstet Anesth.* 2021;45:49-55.

PART II
OBSTETRIC EMERGENCIES

7

Cardiac Arrest

Lior Levy, MD

BACKGROUND

Cardiac arrest in pregnancy is a particularly distressing emergency where we are caring for a patient with altered physiology and her unborn fetus. The U.S. Nationwide Inpatient Sample reports the cardiac arrest rate to be 1 in 12,000 pregnant women admitted for delivery. While survival to discharge of in-hospital arrest in nonpregnant women is shy of 30%, pregnant women fair much better; surviving at ~58%. Given the rate of survival, familiarity with the management of cardiac arrest in pregnancy should have our full attention.[1-3]

Although we are faced with two patients, a mother and infant, the management of cardiac arrest in the parturient focuses on maternal resuscitation regardless of the fetus' gestational age. This is because these measures are often aligned. Since the uterus lacks autoregulation, improving maternal perfusion improves fetal perfusion. Additionally, delivery of the fetus allows for Neonatal Intensive Care Unit (NICU) care for the infant and removal of aortocaval compression in the mom. The improved maternal mortality is why this is now being called a **resuscitative hysterotomy** instead of the older term of *perimortem cesarean delivery*. We should be prepared to perform a resuscitative hysterotomy within **5 minutes** of the arrest to improve the chances of return of spontaneous circulation (ROSC) in the mother.[4,5]

CLINICAL ACTION

Cardiac arrest in pregnancy follows the *same* algorithms and principles in the American Heart Association guidelines but has a few *critical differences*.

Chest compressions, code medications and their doses, as well as defibrillation voltage are identical to the nonpregnant patient.

The differences in the management of a parturient in cardiac arrest are as follows:

- Immediately call an OB code or OB STAT, which would alert anesthesia, obstetricians, and NICU staff alike, as a STAT resuscitative hysterotomy is a likely outcome.
- Continuous manual left uterine displacement (LUD) is essential to minimize aortocaval compression, rendering cardiopulmonary resuscitation ineffective in pregnancy 20 weeks and above. Continuous manual LUD is the best form of LUD in cardiac arrest.
- Favor intravenous access above the diaphragm since venous return is hindered.
- Place lateral defibrillation pad or paddle below breast tissue.
- Before administering a shock, consider removing fetal monitors if it can be done quickly, do not delay shock for that concern. Monitoring fetal heart rate at that time is **NOT** recommended and can divert attention from other resuscitative efforts.

- If the patient is on magnesium, stop the magnesium and intravenous calcium (10 mL of 10% calcium gluconate) should be administered early.
- Pregnant patients are more prone to hypoxia (decreased functional residual capacity and increased oxygen demand). Therefore, oxygenation and airway management should be prioritized higher than in the nonparturient.
- Prepare to face a difficult airway in pregnancy. The first attempt should be by a senior provider with a smaller endotracheal tube (6.5 mm).
- If no return ROSC after 4 minutes, a STAT resuscitative hysterotomy is performed **ON-SITE** if the gravid uterus is estimated or known to be more than 20 weeks (uterus palpable at or above the umbilicus), regardless of fetal viability. The goal is for delivery at 5 minutes postarrest.[6]
- Resuscitative hysterotomy and delivery of the fetus will improve the mother's hemodynamics by relieving aortocaval compression from the gravid uterus and therefore increase the chances for ROSC.
- The patient should not be transported to an operating room for resuscitative hysterotomy; it should be performed at the site of arrest. Transporting the patient has been shown to decrease the quality of chest compression and delay the time until cesarean.
- If the patient is comatose post-ROSC, targeted temperature management should be performed following the same protocols as the nonparturient. If the patient is still pregnant at that time, continuous fetal heart rate monitoring for bradycardia is indicated during the period of targeted temperature management.

ETIOLOGY

While resuscitative efforts are ongoing, it is paramount to evaluate the potential underlying cause of the arrest and formulate a treatment plan. In the United States, leading causes of maternal death are cardiovascular disease and hemorrhage during pregnancy versus infection and hemorrhage in the postpartum period. Below is a list of potential causes of cardiac arrest in the peripartum, group organized alphabetically:

Airway/ventilation: high/total block, airway loss, aspiration, respiratory depression

Accident: trauma, suicide

Bleeding: massive hemorrhage from uterine atony, placenta accrete spectrum, placental abruption, placenta previa, retained product of conception, uterine rupture, cervical laceration, surgical bleeding (could be retroperitoneal), congenital or acquired coagulopathy

Cardiovascular: hypotension, coronary artery dissection, aortic dissection, myocardial infarction, peripartum cardiomyopathy, arrhythmias, valve disease, congenital heart disease

Drugs: overdose of oxytocin, magnesium, opioids, or insulin; medication error, illicit drugs, anaphylaxis reaction, local anesthesia systemic toxicity, transfusion reaction

Embolism: amniotic fluid, air, pulmonary embolus, stroke

Fever: sepsis, infection

General Hs & Ts: hypoxia, hypovolemia, hyperkalemia, hypokalemia and other electrolyte disturbances, hypothermia, hydrogen ion (acidosis), tension pneumothorax, tamponade (cardiac), toxins, thrombosis (coronary and pulmonary)

Hypertension and its complications: including preeclampsia, eclampsia, HELLP (Hemolysis, Elevated Liver enzymes, and Low Platelets) syndrome, intracranial hemorrhage, rupture of liver subcapsular hematoma

References

1. Mhyre JM, Tsen LC, Einav S, Kuklina EV, Leffert LR, Bateman BT. Cardiac arrest during hospitalization for delivery in the United States, 1998-2011. *Anesthesiology*. 2014;120:810-818.

2. Jeejeebhoy FM, Zelop CM, Lipman S, et al. Cardiac arrest in pregnancy: a scientific statement from the American Heart Association. *Circulation*. 2015;132:1747-1773.

3. Merchant RM, Topjian AA, Panchal AR, et al. Part 1: Executive summary: 2020 American Heart Association guidelines for cardiopulmonary resuscitation and emergency cardiovascular care. *Circulation*. 2020;142(16_suppl_2):S337-S357.

4. MacKenzie IZ, Cooke I. What is a reasonable time from decision-to-delivery by caesarean section? Evidence from 415 deliveries. *BJOG*. 2002;109:498-504.

5. Lipman S, Cohen S, Einav S, et al. The Society for Obstetric Anesthesia and Perinatology consensus statement on the management of cardiac arrest in pregnancy. *Anesth Analg*. 2014;118(5):1003-1016.

6. Lipman S, Daniels K, Cohen SE, Carvalho B. Labor room setting compared with the operating room for simulated perimortem cesarean delivery: a randomized controlled trial. *Obstet Gynecol*. 2011;118(5):1090-1094.

8

Amniotic Fluid Embolism

Joan E. Spiegel, MD

BACKGROUND

Amniotic fluid embolism (AFE) incidence is very rare (<1:8000 deliveries) but carries 40% to 80% mortality with at least 50% permanent neurological damage in survivors.[1] Up to 50% of victims will die in the first hour of diagnosis. Approximately 70% occur during labor, 17% during cesarean section, and 11% during postpartum, but can also occur during pregnancy termination or amniocentesis.

The precise etiology of AFE is elusive, with no laboratory tests to confirm diagnosis.[1,2] Clinical pathophysiology stems from maternal infusions of fetal debris (amniotic fluid, meconium, fetal squamous cells, vernix) which causes an abnormal cellular response and anaphylactoid presentation. Systemic immune activation and thrombosis result from the exposure to the numerous immunologically active and prothrombotic substances found in amniotic fluid including platelet-activating factor, interleukins, complement factors, and tumor necrosis factor-alpha. Treatment is supportive.

RISK FACTORS

- Operative vaginal delivery
- Cesarean delivery
- Placenta previa
- Placental abruption
- Meconium
- Induction of labor
- Cervical lacerations
- Induction/augmentation of labor
- Difficult labor or very rapid labor
- Uterine rupture
- Eclampsia
- Polyhydramnios
- Multiple gestation
- Male fetus

DIAGNOSIS[3,4]

AFE is a clinical diagnosis. Clinical symptoms and signs of AFE often occur *suddenly and profoundly*, usually with altered mental status, followed by hypotension and fetal distress in nearly all severe cases (see Table 8-1). May progress rapidly to sudden cardiovascular collapse, cardiac arrest, severe respiratory difficulty and hypoxia, seizures, and disseminated intravascular coagulopathy (DIC). Dysrhythmias are common. Presenting signs and symptoms may occur in any order with variable persistence or severity. In many cases it is a diagnosis of exclusion, relying on autopsy for evidence, or ruling out other disorders (see Table 8-2). Clinical manifestations of AFE are easily remembered as a syndrome of 3Hs: **hypoxia**, **hemodynamic** instability, and **hemorrhage**.

TABLE 8-1 • Signs and Symptoms of AFE	
Signs and Symptoms	**Incidence (%)**
Hypotension	100
Fetal distress	100
Pulmonary edema	93
Cardiac arrest	87
Cyanosis	83
Coagulopathy	83
Dyspnea	49
Seizures	48
Uterine atony	23
Bronchospasm	15

AFE, amniotic fluid embolism.

TABLE 8-2 • Differential Diagnosis in AFE
Differential Diagnosis
Acute hemorrhage
Placental abruption
Uterine rupture
Uterine atony
Eclampsia (not a hypoxic event in most cases)
Cardiomyopathy
High spinal anesthesia (not a cause of severe cardiovascular collapse)
Aspiration
Local anesthetic toxicity (clinical correlation typical)
Pulmonary embolism (not usually accompanied by DIC)
Anaphylaxis (offending agent usually seen)
Septic shock (less dramatic, fever present)

AFE, amniotic fluid embolism; DIC, disseminated intravascular coagulopathy.

PATHOPHYSIOLOGY AND RESPONSE

Clinical response in AFE is conceptualized better when described in phases.

- Phase 1: Entry of fetal material into the maternal circulation causes a systemic inflammatory response with abnormal activation of humoral and immune systems, complement activation, and increased levels of pulmonary vasoconstrictors.
- Phase 2: Acute right ventricular (RV) failure causes hemodynamic collapse via RV infarct or septal displacement into the left ventricle and resultant poor cardiac output. Severe hypoxemia results from a clinical picture similar to pulmonary embolism, i.e., dead space ventilation.
- Phase 3: Left ventricular failure develops with cardiogenic shock.
- Phase 4: DIC may develop with bleeding at surgical and intravenous sites.

CLINICAL PRACTICE AND PROCEDURES (TABLE 8-3)

The medications are used in AFE to stabilize the patient, to decrease the pulmonary vascular resistance, and to improve myocardial contractility. Drugs include norepinephrine, epinephrine, dobutamine, milrinone, inhaled prostacyclin, and inhaled nitric oxide.

TABLE 8-3 • Rapid Response to AFE
• Call for additional help
• Initiate high quality of CPR/ACLS protocols, when appropriate
• Obtain central venous access

• Obtain invasive arterial access for monitoring and sampling:
  • Send arterial blood gas, fibrinogen, and coagulation laboratory tests every 30 minutes
  • Send complete blood count and electrolytes every 60 minutes, at a minimum

• Judicious fluid resuscitation in the setting of right-side heart failure. Consider use of TEE or TTE-guided fluid management
• Initiate pressors to support blood pressure
• Initiate inotropic support early

• Consider additional modalities for decision support:
  • Thromboelastography
  • Transesophageal or transthoracic echocardiogram

• Initiate a massive transfusion protocol
• May consider extracorporeal membrane oxygenation (ECMO)
• Consider ICU transfer when stabilized
• Consider systemic cooling for neuroprotection
• Continually review other etiologies depending on the clinical picture

ACLS, advanced cardiac life support; AFE, amniotic fluid embolism; CPR, cardiopulmonary resuscitation; ICU, intensive care unit; TEE, transesophageal echocardiogram; TTE, transthoracic echocardiogram.

References

1. Pervez S, Seligman K, Carvalho B. Amniotic fluid embolism: update and review. *Curr Opin Anesthesiol.* 2016, 29:288-296.

2. Society for Maternal-Fetal Medicine (SMFM), Pacheco LD, Said G, Hankins GD, et al. Amniotic fluid embolism: diagnosis and management. *Am J Obstet Gynecol.* 2016;215:B16-B24.

3. Gist RS, Stafford IP, Leibowitz AB, Beilin Y. Amniotic fluid embolism. *Anesth Analg.* 2009;108:1599-1602.

4. Metodiev Y, Ramasamy P, Tuffnell D. Amniotic fluid embolism. *Br J Anaesth Education.* 2018;18(8):234-238.

9

Hypertensive Emergency

Patsy J. McGuire, MD

BACKGROUND

Hypertensive disorders of pregnancy complicate nearly 10% of all pregnancies[1-3] and contribute significantly to maternal morbidity and mortality in the United States, most notably in the week following delivery.[4]

Approximately 1% to 2% of all pregnant women will experience a hypertensive emergency during pregnancy or postpartum,[2] defined as ***acute onset blood pressure value $\geq$ 160/110 persisting for 15 minutes or more***.[5] Appropriate and prompt management of hypertension can improve perinatal outcomes and save lives.

COMPLICATIONS

Maternal

• Stroke (hemorrhagic or ischemic)	• HELLP (Hemolysis, Elevated Liver enzymes, and Low Platelet count) syndrome/eclampsia
• Pulmonary edema	• Uteroplacental insufficiency
• Myocardial infarction	• Placental abruption
• Renal failure	• Death

Neonatal

• Intrauterine growth restriction <5th percentile	• Fetal reversed end-diastolic flow

GOALS

- Initiate antihypertensive therapy within 30 to 60 minutes.
- Decrease mean arterial pressure by 20% to 25%.
- Achieve a range of blood pressure (BP) 140-150/90-100 mm Hg.

The overarching goal is maternal stabilization before delivery to avoid maternal end-organ damage. Simultaneous assess for delivery of fetus is also necessary.

CLINICAL MANAGEMENT

Treatment starts with intravenous labetalol or hydralazine, or immediate release oral nifedipine if intravenous (IV) access is not available. Choice is based on physician experience and knowledge of adverse effects.[6]

All algorithms (in tables) start with initial treatment (Tables 9-1 to 9-3), followed by rechecking BP after 10 minutes. If BP control has reached the goal, the treatment may stop bolus medications and initiate a maintenance regimen. If timely relief does not occur, the dose is escalated and emergent consultation with an anesthesiologist, maternal-fetal medicine subspecialist, or critical care subspecialist is recommended.[5] Medications for treating hypertensive crisis are listed in Tables 9-4 and 9-5.

TABLE 9-1 • Start with Hydralazine		
Time (and check BP)	Medication	Dose
Start, time 0	Hydralazine	5-10 mg, IV
At 20 min	Hydralazine	10 mg, IV
Maximum dose is 20 mg per 24 hours		

IV, intravenously.

TABLE 9-2 • Start with Labetalol		
Time (and check BP)	Medication	Dose
Start, time 0	Labetalol	10-20 mg, IV
At 10 min	Labetalol	40 mg, IV
At 20 min	Labetalol	80 mg, IV
At 40 min	Labetalol	80 mg, IV
Maximum dose is 300 mg in 24 hours		

IV, intravenously.

TABLE 9-3 • Start with Nifedipine		
Time (and check BP)	Medication	Dose
Start, time 0	Nifedipine	10 mg, PO
At 20 min	Nifedipine	20 mg, PO
Maximum dose is 180 mg in 24 hours		

PO, orally.

TABLE 9-4 · First-Line Antihypertensive Agents			
	Labetalol	**Hydralazine**	**Nifedipine**
Mechanism	Nonselective β-blocker and α₁-blocker	Direct arteriolar vasodilator	Calcium-channel blocker
Perinatal concerns	Neonatal bradycardia and hypoglycemia	Increased risk for cesarean delivery, abruption, Apgar <7 Neonatal lupus and thrombocytopenia	Fetal distress due to hypotension
Side effects	Bronchoconstriction (severe asthma)	Hypotension, palpitations, tachycardia, headache	Hypotension, palpitations, tachycardia, headache, flushing, peripheral edema
Contraindications	Asthma, advanced AV block, CHF	Mitral valve disease, CAD	Aortic stenosis, CAD

Apgar, Appearance, Pulse, Grimace, Activity, and Respiration; AV block, atrial ventricle block; CAD, coronary artery disease; CHF, congestive heart failure.

TABLE 9-5 · Second-Line Treatment[a]			
	Nicardipine	**Sodium Nitroprusside**	**Esmolol**
Mechanism	Calcium-channel blocker	Nitric oxide releaser	Selective β₁-blocker
Side effects	Headache, dizziness, peripheral edema, flushing, nausea, and vomiting	Cyanide and thiocyanate toxicity; increased ICP	Fetal bradycardia, lightheadedness, bradycardia, peripheral edema, shortness of breath
Contraindications	Severe aortic stenosis	Aortic coarctation, AHF, renal or liver failure, increased ICP	Bradycardia, sick sinus syndrome, AV block, CHF, pulmonary hypertension
Dose (IV)	Initial 5 mg/h Max 15 mg/h	Initial 0.25-0.5 μg/kg/min Max 5 μg/kg/min	Initial 500 μg/kg bolus, then 50 μg/kg/min

[a]Intravenous infusions require close monitoring by an anesthesiologist.
AHF, acute heart failure; AV block, atrial ventricle block; CHF, congestive heart failure; ICP, intracranial pressure.

References

1. Melchiorre K, Thilaganathan B, Giorgione V, Ridder A, Memmo A, Khalil A. Hypertensive disorders of pregnancy and future cardiovascular health. *Front Cardiovasc Med.* 2020;7:5.

2. Too G, Hill J. Hypertensive crisis during pregnancy and postpartum period. *Semin Perinatol.* 2013;37(4):280-287.

3. Vadhera R, Simon M. Hypertensive emergencies in pregnancy. *Clin Obstet Gynecol.* 2014;57(4):797-805.

4. Pregnancy-related deaths: saving women's lives before, during and after delivery. CDC Vital Signs, May 2019.

5. ACOG Committee Opinion No. 767: Emergent therapy for acute-onset, severe hypertension during pregnancy and the postpartum period. *Obstet Gynecol.* 2019;133(2):e174-e180.

6. Duley L, Meher S, Jones L. Drugs for treatment of very high blood pressure during pregnancy. *Cochrane Database Syst Rev.* 2013;2013(7):CD001449.

10

Maternal Early Warning System

Philip E. Hess, MD

The rate of maternal mortality has been increasing in the United States. The maternal mortality rate for 2020 was 23.8/100,000 live births compared with a rate of 17.4 in 2018.[1]

Severe maternal morbidity (SMM) is considered a near miss for maternal mortality if some conditions are not identified and treated. CDC has a consensus list of 21 SMM indicators.[2]

The development of maternal early warning system (MEWS) is to increase the early recognition of changes in the mother's vital signs and clinical conditions leading to prompt evaluation and escalation in the response with the goal of reducing the numbers of women experiencing SMM.[2] A validation cohort study revealed that MEWS showed high specificity, more clinically relevant but with lower sensitivity.[3]

MEWS at Beth Israel Deaconess Medical Center features multidisciplinary collaboration, prompt response with defined actions and guidelines (Fig. 10-1).[4]

Maternal Early Warning Systems (MEWS)

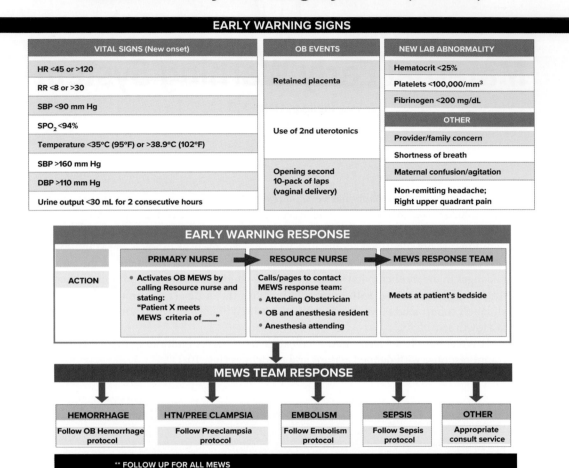

FIGURE 10-1 • Beth Israel Deaconess Medical Center© Maternal Early Warning System. October 2016. (Reproduced with permission from Beth Israel Deaconess Medical Center© Maternal Early Warning System. October 2016.)

References

1. Hoyert DL. Maternal mortality rates in the United States, 2020. National Center for Health Statistics. Centers for Disease Control and Prevention. https://www.cdc.gov/nchs/data/hestat/maternal-mortality/2020/maternal-mortality-rates-2020.htm. Accessed April 2022.

2. Centers for Disease Control and Prevention. How does CDC identify severe maternal morbidity? https://www.cdc.gov/reproductivehealth/maternalinfanthealth/smm/severe-morbidity-ICD.htm. Accessed April 2022.

3. Blumenthal E, Hooshvar N, McQuade M, et al. A validation study of maternal early warning systems: a retrospective cohort study. *Am J Perinatol.* 2019;36(11):1106-1114.

4. Beth Israel Deaconess Medical Center© Maternal Early Warning System. October 2016. Accessed April 2022.

11

Fetal Distress and Intrauterine Resuscitation

Lior Levy, MD

BACKGROUND

Fetal heart rate (FHR) monitoring is the most common obstetric procedure. It is performed to detect fetal hypoperfusion, hypoxia, and acidosis. When the FHR tracing is abnormal, resuscitative measures are taken to increase O_2 delivery to the placenta and improve umbilical blood flow. Ultimately, a cesarean section might be performed if the FHR tracing continues to be concerning. In 2009, American College of Obstetricians and Gynecologists (ACOG) issued a bulletin to streamline the nomenclature and management of FHR monitoring to decrease inter- and intraobserver variability in interpretation.[1,2]

BASICS OF FHR TRACING

- Baseline normal FHR ranges are between 110 and 160 beats per minute (bpm). A sustained change in the heart rate lasting more than 10 minutes constitutes a change in baseline.
- FHR variability is fluctuations in the FHR of two or more cycles (visual regions on the tracing) per minute.
  ○ Moderate variability ranges from 6 to 25 bpm and is considered normal. Moderate variability is a surrogate for the *absence* of metabolic acidemia at the time it is observed.[3]
  ○ Minimal and absent variability raises concern for poor fetal cerebral perfusion. It can also be caused by medications that decrease nervous system activity, such as opioids and magnesium, and is normal during the fetal sleep state.
- Accelerations are abrupt increases in FHR.
  ○ At >32 weeks, an acceleration is 15 beats above baseline, for 15 seconds to 2 minutes.
  ○ At <32 weeks, an acceleration is 10 beats above baseline, for 10 seconds to 2 minutes.
  ○ Presence of accelerations is also typically a sign of fetal well-being, particularly in the antepartum period. Their relevance is less clear intrapartum.
- Decelerations fall into three groups: early, late, and variables. The last two reflect the interruption of oxygen transfer to the fetus at various points along the oxygen delivery pathway.
  ○ **Early decelerations** are characteristically symmetrical to contractions. They are gradual (>30 seconds from onset to nadir) and rarely more than 20 bpm below baseline. They are a normal physiological **vagal reflex to the baby's head** being compressed.

- ○ **Late decelerations** are similar to early decelerations in their gradual nature (>30 seconds from onset to nadir); however, they are delayed in timing. The onset, peak, and end of a late deceleration occur after those of the contraction. They are associated with **uteroplacental insufficiency** and suggest fetal asphyxia. Although not always as sensitive when present alone, they strongly suggest fetal distress when concomitant with decreased or absent FHR variability.
- ○ **Variable decelerations** are abrupt (<30 seconds from onset to nadir) decrease in FHR of 15 or more bpm lasting 15 seconds or more but less than 2 minutes and of variable shapes with each contraction. They are **associated with umbilical cord compression**. When severe and persistent, they are a sign of fetal hypoxia.

INTERPRETATION OF FHR

In 2009, ACOG introduced three categories in which to place FHR tracing to help with management.

Category I:

- Baseline (110 to 160 bpm)
- Moderate variability (6 to 25 bpm)
- No late or variable decelerations
- Accelerations present or not
- Early deceleration present or not

Category II:

- All tracings not in category I or III

Category III:

- ABSENT VARIABILITY AND any of:
  - ○ Recurrent late decelerations
  - ○ Recurrent variable decelerations
  - ○ Bradycardia
- OR sinusoidal

While category I generally predicts intact fetal health and requires no further action, category II cannot adequately predict normal or abnormal acid-base status. It requires re-evaluation, continued surveillance, and may compel intrauterine resuscitative measures to address possible ongoing fetal distress. Category III is associated with abnormal fetal acid-based status and hypoxia. It requires intrauterine measures and possibly a cesarean delivery if these do not improve the tracing.

CLINICAL ACTIONS

When the obstetric team identifies a concerning FHR tracing, the anesthesia team presents to the bedside. Intrauterine resuscitations are initiated to improve placental perfusion and restore a reassuring FHR tracing.[2]

Maternal positioning

- Left uterine displacement to decrease aortocaval compression and improve maternal hemodynamics and uteroplacental blood flow
- Try left, right, and all-fours positions to relieve pressure on main vessels

Maternal hemodynamics and oxygenation
• Correct maternal hypotension • Intravenous fluids • Vasopressors as needed (phenylephrine preferred) • Supplemental O_2 to be used only to correct maternal hypoxemia ($SpO_2 < 94\%$). Empirical use of O_2 to improve FHT is not evidence-based and is no longer in practice[4]
Tocolysis
In the presence of uterine tachysystole (sustained uterine contraction leading to non-reassuring FHR tracing): • Administer intravenous (IV) fluids. • Stop oxytocin administration. • Administer terbutaline 250 µg subcutaneously. • No evidence to use tocolytics unless tachysystole (>5 contractions in 10 minutes averaged over 30-minute period) or uterine hypertonus (single contraction lasting >2 minutes) is present.
Progression of labor
• Conduct cervical exam to check for rapid cervical dilation, descent of fetal head, or umbilical cord prolapse. • In trial of labor after cesarean (TOLAC) patients, **consider uterine rupture** (abdominal pain). • In the presence of variable decelerations, uterine amnioinfusion with saline should be considered (bolus or continuous).
The anesthesia team should head to the bedside and consider neuraxial placement or evaluate that the current labor epidural is in place and has an appropriate level in case of imminent cesarean delivery. It is judicious to be prepared with a chloroprocaine vial and an empty syringe if an emergent cesarean delivery is called.

LIMITS OF FHR MONITORING

The efficacy of FHR is based on its ability to decrease complications such as poor neonatal neurological outcome and intrapartum death, while minimizing the rate of operative deliveries. The rate of cesarean delivery and operative vaginal delivery is undoubtedly higher. Retrospective studies associate continuous FHR monitoring with decreased perinatal complications and neonatal deaths. Meta-analysis of prospective studies on the other hand have only shown that continuous FHR monitoring decreases the rate of neonatal seizures and the incidence of Apgar scores <4 at 1 minute. The rate of cerebral palsy has remained unchanged, which might be multifactorial (neurological injury might not happen intrapartum, more and more severely premature infants survive, etc.). There also does not seem to be a clear advantage to continuous versus intermittent FHR monitoring, which is in agreement with ACOG recommendation of either being acceptable. The poor positive predictive value of FHR monitoring in determining negative fetal outcome has not deterred most obstetricians to depend on it and as anesthesiologists we must be ready to participate in the management of patients with non-reassuring fetal status.

References

1. Practice Bulletin No. 116: Management of intrapartum fetal heart rate tracings. *Obstet Gynecol.* November 2010;116(5):1232-1240.

2. Garite TJ, Simpson KR. Intrauterine resuscitation during labor. *Clin Obstet Gynecol.* 2011;54(1):28-39.

3. Williams KP, Galerneau F. Intrapartum fetal heart rate patterns in the prediction of neonatal acidemia. *Am J Obstet Gynecol.* 2003;188:820-823.

4. Raghuraman N, Temming LA, Doering MM, et al. Maternal oxygen supplementation compared with room air for intrauterine resuscitation: a systematic review and meta-analysis. *JAMA Pediatr.* 2021;175(4):368-376.

12

Shoulder Dystocia, Cord Prolapse, Uterine Inversion, Uterine Rupture

Justin K. Stiles, MD

SHOULDER DYSTOCIA[1]

Incidences:	5-9% if fetal weights of 4000-4500 g
	14-21% if fetal weights of 4500-5000 g
	American College of Obstetricians and Gynecologists (ACOG) recommends cesarean delivery for 5000 g without diabetes, 4500 g with diabetes. However, diagnosis of macrosomia is imprecise.
Diagnosis:	Turtle sign—Retraction of head against maternal perineum immediately after delivery of the head. Or resistance of delivery of anterior shoulder with usual traction to fetal head.

Risk Factors

Maternal

Abnormal pelvic anatomy
Gestational or pregestational diabetes
Previous shoulder dystocia
Short stature (<60 in)
Obese (>200 lbs)
Previous large infant (>4000 g)
Excessive weight gain

Fetal

Suspected macrosomia

Labor

Operative vaginal delivery
Protracted active phase
Prolonged second stage
Precipitous labor

Be CALM

Breathe, do not push
Elevate legs, McRoberts position (knee/chest supine)
Call for help
Apply suprapubic NOT fundal pressure
Enlarge vaginal opening with episiotomy
Maneuvers to rotate baby to deliver posterior arm

Extraordinary Maneuvers

Fracture fetal clavicle
Zavenelli maneuver—cephalic replacement for cesarean delivery
Symphysiotomy

Complications

Maternal

Postpartum hemorrhage
Rectovaginal fistula
Symphysial separation or diathesis with or without femoral neuropathy
Third to fourth degree tear or episiotomy
Uterine rupture

Fetal

Brachial plexus injury
Clavicle or humeral fracture
Fetal hypoxia with or without permanent neurological injury
Fetal death

UMBILICAL CORD PROLAPSE

Sudden and significant cord compression leads to immediate and sustained fetal bradycardia.

Risk Factors

Premature rupture of membrane (PROM), iatrogenic ROM with presenting part not well applied
   to cervix
Vaginal delivery of twins
Vaginal delivery of footling breech

Intervention

Manual elevation of fetal head off cervix until emergent cesarean delivery.

UTERINE INVERSION

Uterus turns itself inside out with the fundus passing through the cervix into the vagina leading
to severe and sudden postpartum hemorrhage, significant discomfort, and severe nausea and
vomiting.

Risk Factors

Excess traction on cord applied to facilitate delivery of placenta, or excess fundal pressure on a relaxed uterus

About 1 in 2000 to 1 in 6400 vaginal deliveries

Fundal implantation of uterus is potential risk

Higher risk in primigravida

Treatment

Manually pushing the fundus back through the cervix, which should be done immediately before cervical constriction. Delay delivery of placenta if it still attaches to the uterus to limit additional bleeding while maintaining an elevated concern for abnormal placentation.

Uterine relaxation/cervical dilation can be facilitated with tocolytics: volatile anesthesia, terbutaline (250 µg, subcutaneously) or nitroglycerin (50-100 µg, IV).

After uterine inversion is resolved, immediately provide uterotonics and resuscitation of patient.

UTERINE RUPTURE

Uterine rupture, separation of the unscarred uterine muscle, or a previous cesarean section scar can occur before or during labor resulting in massive hemorrhage.

Risk Factors

Prior cesarean section or uterine surgery

Use of prostaglandins for cervical ripening during a trial of labor after cesarean

Effect of oxytocin on the risk of rupture remains unclear

Still possible without prior uterine scar

Diagnosis

Fetal heart rate abnormalities

Vaginal bleeding

Maternal hypovolemia

Significant pain refractory to analgesic boluses

Reverse of station

Obstetric Management

If diagnosis is made after delivery, a watchful waiting approach is possible unless hematologic or hemodynamic decompensation occurs. If during labor, perform an exploratory laparotomy with delivery of fetus and repair of defect with possible hysterectomy.

Reference

1. Datta S, ed. *Anesthetic and Obstetric Management of High-Risk Pregnancy*. 3rd ed. New York: Springer-Verlag; 2004.

13

Postpartum Hemorrhage and Placenta Accreta Spectrum

Philip E. Hess, MD

BACKGROUND

Postpartum hemorrhage (PPH) is one of the leading causes of severe maternal morbidity and mortality worldwide and in the United States.[1,2] Cesarean delivery rate has increased significantly in the last three decades. Consequently, the incidence of placenta accreta spectrum (PAS) has also increased.[3]

Many education and safety resources have been developed for PPH and have evolved into Obstetric Hemorrhage Bundles. Here are some additional resources for PPH information:

- The Alliance for Innovation on Maternal Health (AIM)—Patient Safety Bundles: Obstetric Hemorrhage[4]
- California Maternal Quality Care Collaborative (CMQCC)[5]—OB Hemorrhage Toolkit v3.0
- The American College of Obstetricians and Gynecologists (ACOG)—Postpartum Hemorrhage,[6] Practice bulletin number 183

The Obstetric Hemorrhage Bundle at Beth Israel Deaconess Medical Center (BIDMC) emphasizes the following aspects (**3Rs**):

- **R**eadiness for PPH: mandatory simulation training course, online modules, in-person workshop, PPH cart, quantitative blood loss (QBL), uterotonics (Chapter 5 "Uterotonics")
- **R**ecognition of PPH in a timely fashion: evaluation tool for obstetric hemorrhage risk (Chapter 34 "Evaluation of Hemorrhage Risks")
- **R**esponse to PPH: BIDMC Massive Transfusion Protocol, guidelines of active management of the third stage of labor, guidelines for uterotonics use for cesarean delivery (Chapter 4 "Oxytocin"), guidelines for obstetric hemorrhage, and guidelines for escalating notification (Chapter 53 "Postanesthetic Care") and rapid response team for PPH

The New England Center for Placental Disorders at BIDMC is a unique and robust multidisciplinary program for treating patients with PAS disorders. It draws patients from around the region, country, and world. Highly efficient, cooperative, and coordinated teams are the cornerstones of this very successful program.

This chapter will outline some clinical pearls for anesthesiologists who manage scheduled and urgent PAS cases. The latter is the most challenging case for obstetric anesthesiologists. Detailed guidelines and extensive training for the entire obstetric anesthesia team are the preconditions for the success.

PREPARATION FOR PAS CASES

All obstetric anesthesiologists should follow the *same protocol* for preparing the operating room for PAS cases. The protocol was developed using an *iterative improvement technique*—after every PAS surgery, the team was interviewed in a structured manner to optimize workflow and logistics. Consistent preparation among the providers can ensure efficient teamwork, especially in a time-limited situation.

BEFORE THE SURGERY

- Anesthesia consult: review the medical history, airway exam, discuss the anesthetic plans, need for blood transfusion, and consent
- Multidisciplinary meeting: attended by Maternal-Fetal Medicine, Obstetric Anesthesia, Nursing, Blood Bank, Urology, Gynecology-Oncology (backups), Neonatal ICU, and Perfusionist
- Patient education

ANESTHETIC OPERATING ROOM PREPARATION

Right Side of Bed

Arterial line transducer and zeroed
Infusion pump with large phenylephrine syringe (240 µg/mL), primed
Infusion pump with large norepinephrine syringe (32 µg/mL), not primed
Infusion pump with large epinephrine syringe (8 µg/mL), not primed
PlasmaLyte with blood IV tubing through Ranger warmer
Lactated Ringer's microdrip tubing through multiple-port connector (to 20G IV on the right arm)

Left Side of Bed

Belmont rapid infuser, PlasmaLyte primed
Second Ranger's fluid warmer with PlasmaLyte with blood tubing

Extra Equipment

Ultrasound machine.
McGrath or Glidescope.*
Red hemorrhage folder contains all necessary paperwork.*
Pre-fill arterial blood gas (ABG) and laboratory paperwork, patient labels prepped (name, phone extension, date).
Super-STAT stickers for quick laboratory process.*
Bair Hugger ×2 (underbody and upper).*
Activate pulse pressure variation (PPV) on arterial line waveform on Philip's monitor.
Take head segment off the top of the operating table and put on the foot end for lithotomy position.
Ensure rapid infusion catheter (RIC) kit and central line (MAC line) kit are available in the emergency cart.*

*Items are already located in the operating room.

PHARMACY

From Main Omnicell on Labor and Delivery:

1 g calcium chloride, 5 doses
50 mL phenylephrine, norepinephrine, and epinephrine syringes
    From the Omnicell in the operating room:
Confirm carboprost and methylergonovine available in operating room fridge (two of each)
2 g premixed cefazolin, 2 doses
1 g tranexamic acid, dilute in 10 mL

REMINDER

Re-dose cefazolin with 1.5 L blood loss
1 g tranexamic acid intravenously after delivery
Re-dose tranexamic acid if excessive bleeding, consider infusion

FROM BLOOD BANK

Cooler with 4 units of packed red blood cell, 2 units of fresh frozen plasma to start
Two-person check all blood products before the case
Activate massive transfusion protocol, as needed
Change ratio to 1:1 if fibrinogen <300 mg/dL

DURING CASE

Move regional cart and other equipment out of room after use (create space)
Move fetal monitor out of room after the case started
Move cystoscope tower out of room when done
Make sure nursing is prepared for quantitative blood loss measurement

PATIENT PREPARATION

16G or 14G peripheral IV (×2)
Radial arterial line (better on right but not important)
20G IV for infusions (good vein so can be changed for RIC in the operating room)
Discuss the anesthetic plan with the patient.

EMERGENCY PHONE NUMBERS

Blood bank
Blood runner: usually a nurse; all communication with blood bank is through the blood
    runner ONLY
Main Pharmacy
STAT laboratory
Perfusionist: pager number (should put # on board if she/he steps out)

ANESTHETIC MANAGEMENT FOR PAS CASE

The anesthetic plan is tailored to meet individual patient's need. In BIDMC, a great majority of PAS cases have been performed comfortably under combined spinal and epidural anesthesia.

Combined Spinal and Epidural (CSE)

- The preferred choice. The benefits of CSE include quick onset, dense block for patient comfort, the ability to be extended if the surgery is prolonged, awake mother to experience childbirth, minimal placental transfer of medications, and the ability to administer neuraxial morphine for quality postoperative analgesia. Can supplement with light sedation for anxious patients or longer surgery.
- May need to be converted to general anesthesia because of prolonged surgery, discomfort from uterine manipulation, patient anxiety, and potential difficulty with intubation after resuscitation. If the need to convert is anticipated, consider early general anesthesia.

Epidural

- Same pros and cons as CSE except slower onset. In patients with cardiac comorbidities, slow sympathectomy is desired (Chapter 15 "Cardiac Diseases").

General Anesthesia

- General anesthesia is rarely the first choice.
- Indications: difficult airway, absolute contraindications to neuraxial anesthesia, patient's request.

Intraoperative Management

See Fig. 13-1. They are posted in each operating room.

References

1. Berg CJ, Chang J, Callaghan WM, Whitehead SJ. Pregnancy-related mortality in the United States, 1991-1997. *Obstet Gynecol.* 2003;101:289-296.
2. Bateman BT, Berman MF, Riley LE, Leffert LR. The epidemiology of postpartum hemorrhage in a large, nationwide sample of deliveries. *Anesth Analg.* 2010;110:1368-1373.
3. Solheim KN, Esakoff TF, Little SE, et al. The effect of cesarean delivery rates on the future incidence of placenta previa, placenta accreta, and maternal mortality. *I Matern Fetal Neonatal Med.* 2011;24(11):1341-1346.
4. Alliance for Innovation on Maternal Health (AIM). The Obstetric hemorrhage bundle. https://safehealthcareforeverywoman.org/aim/patient-safety-bundles/maternal-safety-bundles/obstetric-hemorrahage-patient-safety-bundle-2/.
5. California Maternal Quality Care Collaborative (CMQCC). OB Hemorrhage Toolkit, V 3.0 https://www.cmqcc.org/resources-tool-kits/toolkits/ob-hemorrhage-toolkit.
6. The American College of Obstetricians and Gynecologists (ACOG). Postpartum hemorrhage. Practice bulletin number 183. October 2017. https://www.acog.org/clinical/clinical-guidance/practice-bulletin/articles/2017/10/postpartum-hemorrhage.

Transfusion Guidelines

Additional Monitoring	Medications	Laboratory Test	Transfusion
□ Arterial line □ PPV—validated in nonintubated patients (*Anesth Analg.* 2015; 120:76-84) □ Base excess—with prognostic value (Colella et al. SOAP Annual Meeting, 2018) □ Lactic acid □ Quantitative blood loss (QBL) □ Temperature □ Urine output □ Ultrasound: volume and contractility assessment	□ Uterotonics □ Tranexamic acid 1 g □ Cefazolin: 2 g q4h, repeat when blood loss ≥1500 mL □ CaCl$_2$, IV: when ionized calcium is low, or with 3rd set of packed red blood cell/fresh frozen plasma	Labs sent q30 min for massive PPH: □ PT/PTT/INR □ Fibrinogen □ Blood gas with pH, base excess, potassium, ionized calcium, hematocrit, Lactic acid Labs sent q60 min for massive PPH: □ CBC Note: Consider TEG if laboratory results delayed or not matching clinical picture	□ Notify the resource nurse □ Activate Massive Blood Transfusion Protocol □ Start 1:1:2, switch to 1:1:1 when coagulation affected □ Designate a Blood Bank runner □ Designate a person to run Belmont □ Cell saver—call perfusion □ Transfusion guidelines (see below)

Red Blood Cell	Fresh Frozen Plasma	Cryoprecipitate	Crystalloid	Platelet
PPV >10 Hematocrit <27% Fibrinogen >3 g/L	PPV >10 Hematocrit >27% Fibrinogen <3 g/L	PPV <10 Hematocrit >27% Fibrinogen <2 g/L	PPV >10 Hematocrit >27% Fibrinogen >3 g/L	<50,000/mm^3 OR <75,000/mm^3 with active uncontrolled bleeding

PPV, pulse pressure variation; TEG, thromboelastography.

FIGURE 13-1 • Postpartum hemorrhage workflow.

PART III

HIGH-RISK OBSTETRICS

14

Preeclampsia and Eclampsia

Erin J. Ciampa, MD, PhD

PATHOPHYSIOLOGY AND CLINICAL PRESENTATION OF PREECLAMPSIA

- Multisystem disease attributable to endothelial dysfunction.
- Preeclampsia is clinically defined by **new onset** (after 20 weeks of gestation) of **hypertension** (systolic blood pressure [SBP] ≥140 mm Hg or diastolic blood pressure [DBP] ≥90 mm Hg) and **proteinuria**. Preeclampsia can also be diagnosed in the absence of proteinuria, if one or more **systemic manifestations** are present (see Table 14-1).[1]
- Preeclampsia is said to have severe features if blood pressure is high, i.e., SBP ≥160 mm Hg or DBP ≥110 mm Hg, or with the presence of one or more **systemic manifestations** (see below).[1]
- Early onset (<34 weeks gestational age) preeclampsia typically carries greater risk of maternal/fetal complications (see Table 14-2).
- Occurrence of seizures not attributable to any other cause = eclampsia (seizure may be a presenting sign).

TABLE 14-1 • Systemic Manifestations of Preeclampsia

Feature	Clinical Criteria
Proteinuria	>300 mg over 24 hours, or protein:creatinine ratio >0.3
Thrombocytopenia	<100,000/μL
Renal insufficiency	Serum creatinine >1.1 mg/dL, or doubling from baseline
Liver dysfunction	Transaminases >2× baseline
Pulmonary edema	
Cerebral symptoms	Unexplained headache not responsive to medical treatment, or visual disturbance

TABLE 14-2 • Additional Potential Complications

Cardiomyopathy	Pulmonary edema
Myocardial infarction	Seizure
Intracranial hemorrhage	Retinal injury
Renal failure	Coagulopathy
Hepatic injury/rupture	Liver subcapsular bleeding
Fetal growth restriction	Placental abruption

CLINICAL MANAGEMENT

Obstetric Decision-Making Examples[1]

Preeclampsia **without severe features**: continued monitoring and expectant management until 37 weeks of gestational age, then induction of labor (or cesarean delivery if obstetric indication is present).

Preeclampsia **with severe features**:

$\geq$34 weeks of gestational age, delivery is recommended after maternal stabilization.

<34 weeks of gestational age with stable maternal and fetal condition, expectant management may be considered.

<34 weeks of gestational age with any clinical instability, delivery soon after maternal stabilization.

Intrapartum Management Cornerstones

1. Blood pressure (BP) monitoring and treatment:
   - At least once per hour predelivery
   - Automated BP cuff may underestimate actual BP. Check with manual cuff. Place arterial line for monitoring if divergent.
   - Target SBP <160 mm Hg, DBP <110 mm Hg. Be aware that excessive lowering BP can cause a rapid decrease in uteroplacental perfusion.
   - First-line therapy: labetalol; second-line: hydralazine, nifedipine.
2. Seizure prophylaxis[2]:
   - Magnesium sulfate 4 to 6 g intravenous bolus followed by 1 to 2 g/h infusion (renally cleared; reduce dose if renal insufficiency).
   - Target range: 5 to 9 mg/dL.
   - Signs of toxicity: loss of deep tendon reflexes (9.6-12 mg/dL), hypotension, respiratory depression (12-18 mg/dL), hypoxia, EKG changes, and cardiac arrest (24-30 mg/dL).
   - Treatment of magnesium toxicity: $CaCl_2$ intravenously.
3. Mild fluid restriction (<1 mL/kg/h maintenance during induction of labor and labor) and urine output monitoring.
4. Eclamptic seizure treatment:
   - First-line: magnesium sulfate (4 g bolus over 5 minutes, then 1 g/h infusion).
   - Adjuncts: benzodiazepines, phenytoin.
   - Consider alternative causes (local anesthetics systemic toxicity, electrolyte derangement, epilepsy, severe rigor from large dose of misoprostol).
   - Fetal bradycardia is common due to temporary hypoxemia and hypercarbia; it is not necessarily an indication for emergent cesarean delivery.

Anesthesia Considerations[3]

1. Check platelets prior to neuraxial in any patient with hypertension.
2. General anesthesia is less desirable due to the risk of severe hypertension/cerebral hemorrhage with intubation/extubation and possible difficult intubation.
3. Spinal anesthesia for cesarean delivery is not contraindicated.
4. Consider early epidural for labor analgesia if platelet count is trending down.
5. Fluid restriction: preload/co-load not necessary in patients with preeclampsia; judicious crystalloid use in cesarean delivery.
6. Beware of magnesium toxicity, especially if renal impairment.

7. Beware of high risk of postpartum hemorrhage.
8. Uterotonic agents: avoid methergine. Consider tranexamic acid and calcium chloride in addition to regular uterotonic agents.
9. Avoid ketorolac if renal insufficiency.

References

1. ACOG Practice Bulletin no. 222: Gestational hypertension and preeclampsia. *Obstet Gynecol*. 2020;135(6):e237-e260.
2. The Magpie Trial Collaborative Group. Magnesium sulphate prevented eclampsia in women with pre-eclampsia. *Lancet*. 2002;359:1877-1890.
3. Leffert L. What's new in obstetric anesthesia? Focus on preeclampsia. *Int J Obstet Anesth*. 2015;24(3):264-271.

15

Cardiac Diseases

Philip E. Hess, MD

BACKGROUND

Pregnancy in women with heart diseases carries significant risks to the mother and her fetus. Cardiovascular conditions are the leading cause of maternal death in the United States.[1] The number of women with cardiac disorders/conditions in pregnancy is increasing in the United States, due to:

- Increased survival in patients with congenital heart diseases allowing these women to reach childbearing age.
- The incidence of rheumatic valvular diseases is trending down, rheumatic:congenital 25:1 is now 3:1, and most of rheumatic valvular diseases is mitral stenosis (90%).[2]
- Increasing incidence of coronary artery disease (CAD) because of delayed childbearing age.
- Smoking and drug use.

The anesthesiologists can make significant contribution in the monitoring and management of pregnant women with heart diseases to improve maternal outcomes. We emphasize that epidural analgesia and anesthesia must be modified and individualized to the cardiac patients and minimize to the maximum the hemodynamic changes from analgesia and anesthesia. The decision of delivery model, cardiology care, invasive intervention, and surgical management options are beyond the scope of the current chapter.

HEART DISEASES IN PREGNANCY

High-risk conditions—these conditions are most affected by the physiologic changes during pregnancy (Box 15-1):

- Pulmonary hypertension, primary and secondary
- Eisenmenger syndrome
- Complex congenital heart diseases
- Aortic dilation/dissection—most commonly due to Marfan syndrome and congenital connective tissue diseases
- Severe aortic valve stenosis—most commonly due to bicuspid valves, other causes include Marfan syndrome
- Severe mitral valve stenosis
- Ventricle dysfunction
- Peripartum cardiomyopathy[3]

BOX 15-1 • Predictors of Adverse Cardiac Events[4,5]

The **modified CARPREG risk score** is based on a point-value to estimate the potential of an adverse cardiac event. One point is an assessed risk of 5% or less, two or three points = 10% to 15%, the risk at four points is over 20%, and a patient with greater than four points has more than a 40% chance of a major adverse event. Points are assigned based on the woman's current status and the type of disease.

Current status:

NYHA class III-IV adds three points:

- The presence of maternal cyanosis equates to NYHA III.
- Prior major cardiac event or serious arrhythmia also is valued at three points.
- If a woman has had no cardiac work-up prior to pregnancy or the first assessment is in late pregnancy—each adds one point.

Type of disease:

A woman having a mechanical heart valve is worth three points.

Other high-risk cardiac conditions are worth two points, including ventricular dysfunction, left-sided valves disease or outflow obstruction, pulmonary hypertension (systolic pressure $\geq$70 mm Hg), coronary artery disease, or aortopathy (e.g., ascending aortic dilation of 4.0 cm).

CARPREG, Canadian cardiac disease in pregnancy; LVOT, left ventricular outflow tract; NYHA, New York Heart Association functional class.

Variable-risk conditions:

- Mitral valve prolapse—most common cardiac disorder among women of childbearing age, or a congenital condition due to redundant leaflets
- Arrhythmias
- Hypertrophic cardiomyopathy
- CAD—often vasospastic disease or dissection

Lower-risk conditions (usually)—these conditions can better tolerate the physiologic changes in pregnancy:

- Mitral regurgitation
- Aortic regurgitation

MULTIDISCIPLINARY CARDIO-OBSTETRIC TEAM[5,6]

- All obstetric providers perform a basic screening of cardiac conditions on a routine basis. Of note, many cardiac disease–related symptoms will overlap with some symptoms and signs related to late pregnancy, such as tachycardia, shortness of breath, edema, and even arrhythmia.
- Refer the pregnant woman with cardiac diseases/conditions to maternal-fetal medicine (MFM). Maintain a communication pathway for transfers from community hospitals.
- The Beth Israel Deaconess Medical Center has established a multidisciplinary "Cardio-Obstetric Team" embracing healthcare providers from MFM, obstetrics, cardiology, obstetric anesthesia, and nursing. Cardiologists are specialized in pregnant women with cardiac diseases. The "Cardio-Obstetric Team" begins communication as early as the first or second trimester and maintains communication throughout labor and postpartum period. Scheduled conferences at regular interval allows review of all potential cases and coordinated care for each individual patient.
- Availability of intensive care unit.

GOALS OF ANESTHETIC MANAGEMENT

- Tailor the anesthetic plan on individual basis.
- Maintain maternal cardiac output and vital signs near baseline—the most susceptible component is *preload.*
- Avoid sympathetic stress—massive increase in physical stress during painful labor and delivery, sympathetic surge during endotracheal intubation/extubation.
- Avoid increased intrathoracic pressure—mechanical ventilation with large tidal volume during general anesthesia, prolonged second stage Valsalva maneuvers. A passive second stage of labor may be more appropriate for some patients.
- Avoid increasing pulmonary vascular resistance—avoid hypercarbia, hypoxemia, hypothermia, and acidosis.
- Tolerate postdelivery volume expansion, especially immediately after delivery with abrupt rise in intravascular volume due to autotransfusion.
- Prevent excessive blood loss during labor—associated with maternal tachycardia and decreased stroke volume—early transfusion may be indicated.
- Arterial line for NYHA 3 or 4, or high-risk patients, telemetry monitoring, pulse oximetry for pulmonary hypertension, and Eisenmenger syndrome.
- Uterotonics—use with caution (stated in Table 15-1).

REGIONAL VERSUS GENERAL ANESTHESIA

Both general and regional anesthesia are used for the care of the pregnant woman with cardiac disease and assessing the pros and cons may help formulate a plan. We typically *favor* the use of epidural analgesia/anesthesia for both labor and cesarean due to the ability to slow the onset of sympathectomy and functionally block cardiovascular stress. (See Table 15-2.)

ANESTHETIC MANAGEMENT FOR CARDIAC CESAREAN DELIVERY

Goals and Targets

- Reduce stress during surgery.
- Maintain fetal perfusion.
- Maintain maternal blood pressure and cardiac output.
- Slow onset sympathectomy.
- Dense blockade during surgery.

TABLE 15-1 • Uterotonics Use	
Uterotonics	**Contraindications**
Oxytocin	No contraindication; avoid large dose bolus
Carboprost	Use with caution in pulmonary hypertension
Methylergonovine	Use with caution with obstructive lesions, CAD, pulmonary hypertension
Misoprostol	Large dose may cause severe rigors and fever (increase in oxygen demand)

TABLE 15-2 • Comparison of Regional Anesthesia Versus General Anesthesia

Regional Analgesia/Anesthesia	General Anesthesia
Pros	*Pros*
Labor analgesia can offload the cardiovascular stress during contractions	Controllable sympathectomy
Neuraxial anesthesia prevents cardiovascular stress	Very low failure rate
Provides high-quality postoperative analgesia	
Avoids airway intervention	
Spontaneous ventilation	
Slow onset epidural—controlled sympathetic loss	
Cons	*Cons*
Possible hemodynamic instability during induction	Poor adrenergic control related to laryngoscopy and strenuous coughing during extubation
Rapid sympathectomy—loss of preload, decreased systemic vascular resistance, reflex increase in heart rate	Increased intrathoracic pressure during ventilation
Labor analgesia failure can increase morbidity	High dose of narcotics could lead to prolonged ventilation and neonatal sedation
Anticoagulation is a contraindication	Less effective postoperative pain control
	Inhalation agents can cause decreased preload and myocardial depression

Preparation

Phenylephrine infusion in line.
Norepinephrine (obstructive lesions, cardiomyopathy).
Nitroglycerin (mitral stenosis, coronary disease).
Minimize fluid administration.
Arterial line, central venous line, and pulmonary artery catheter, as needed.

Epidural Anesthesia

This is intended as a general pathway, which can be modified as needed.
Place an epidural catheter as per usual:

- May use spinal needle to ensure epidural space and midline insertion.
- NO test dose for obstructive lesion or arrhythmia (epinephrine may be deleterious).

Examples of titrated dosing:

- 0.5% bupivacaine, 2 mL given every 5 minutes epidurally.
- 50 μg fentanyl on third dose.
- Test level after fifth dose:
  - Assess for sensory changes in feet.
  - Level check to cold sensation.
- After 20 mL bolus, wait for T10 level.

- Fentanyl 50 µg when T10 level is achieved.
- May use 2% lidocaine with bicarbonate (no epinephrine) after T6 level is achieved

After Delivery

Use uterotonics use with caution (Table 15-1).
Autotransfusion management for mitral stenosis or at risk for acute heart failure:

- Use 10 mg furosemide intravenously.
- Use nitroglycerin infusion titrated to symptoms or central venous pressure or pulmonary pressures.
- Consider phlebotomy for acute decompression of volume overload (obtain a phlebotomy bag from blood bank—need central line).

LABOR EPIDURAL ANALGESIA FOR CARDIAC VAGINAL DELIVERY

Goals and Targets

- Reduce stress during labor and expulsion.
- Maintain fetal perfusion.
- Maintain maternal blood pressure and cardiac output.
- *Slow onset sympathectomy*—key component of cardiac epidural (attached protocol for titration of epidural analgesia).
- Early epidural to allow time to titration of epidural analgesia.
- Dense blockade during second stage of labor.
- Passive second stage—forceps or vacuum delivery.

  This is intended as a general pathway, which can be modified as needed.

Epidural Analgesia

Place an epidural catheter as per usual.

- May use spinal needle to ensure epidural space and midline insertion.
- If in painful labor, may give intrathecal 25 µg fentanyl, NO bupivacaine (no effect on preload).
- NO test dose (epinephrine may be deleterious).
- Aspirate catheter prior to all injections.
- No patient controlled epidural analgesia.
- No programmed intermittent epidural bolus.
- Begin infusion of 0.04% bupivacaine with fentanyl 1.7 µg/mL at 15 mL/h.
  - NO bolus to avoid hypotension.
  - After 1 hour, check for sensory change.
  - Usually tingling in both feet and/or sensory level to cold.
- May change to 0.0625% bupivacaine with fentanyl after 1 to 2 hours infusion.
- Maintain infusion rate at 15 mL/h.
- Increase bupivacaine concentration every 2 hours and slowly to 0.08%, 0.125%, 0.1875%, as needed, to have dense sacral level (Box 15-2).

  After sympathectomy has been achieved additional local anesthetic should not cause a significant change in blood pressure.

- It is reasonable to use 2% lidocaine or 3% chloroprocaine for cesarean delivery.

BOX 15-2 • Titration of Cardiac Epidural Analgesia

1. **Bupivacaine 0.04%, fentanyl 1.7 µg/mL**
   a. Pre-made bupivacaine/fentanyl bag from pharmacy
   b. No epinephrine added
2. **Bupivacaine 0.0625%, fentanyl 1.7 µg/mL**
   a. Bupivacaine 0.25%: 15 mL
   b. Fentanyl 50 µg/mL: 2 mL
   c. PF normal saline: 43 mL
   Total 60 mL
   PF: preservative free
3. **Bupivacaine 0.08%, fentanyl 1.7 µg/mL**
   a. Bupivacaine 0.25%: 19 mL
   b. Fentanyl 50 µg/mL: 2 mL
   c. PF normal saline: 39 mL
   Total 60 mL
4. **Bupivacaine 0.125%, fentanyl 1.7 µg/mL**
   a. Bupivacaine 0.25%: 30 mL
   b. Fentanyl 50 µg/mL: 2 mL
   c. PF normal saline: 28 mL
   Total 60 mL
5. **Bupivacaine 0.1875%, fentanyl 1.7 µg/mL**
   a. Bupivacaine 0.25%: 112.5 mL
   b. Fentanyl 50 µg/mL: 5 mL
   c. PF normal saline: 32.5 mL
   Total 150 mL

References

1. CDC. Pregnancy mortality surveillance system. Causes of pregnancy-related deaths. https://www.cdc.gov/reproductivehealth/maternal-mortality/pregnancy-mortality-surveillance-system.htm. Accessed April 2022.

2. Mangano DT. Anesthesia for the pregnant cardiac patient. In: Hughes SC, Levinson G, Rosen MA, eds. *Shnider and Levinson's Anesthesia for Obstetrics*. 4th ed. Philadelphia, PA: Lippincott Williams & Wilkins; 2002:455-486.

3. Patten IS, Rana S, Shahul S, et al. Cardiac angiogenic imbalance leads to peripartum cardiomyopathy. *Nature*. 2012;485:333-338.

4. Silversides CK, Grewal J, Mason J, et al. Pregnancy outcomes in women with heart disease. The CARPREG II study. *J Am Coll Cardiol*. 2018;71:2419-2430.

5. Canobbio MM, Warnes CA, Aboulhosn J, et al. Management of pregnancy in patients with complex congenital heart disease. A scientific statement for healthcare professionals from the American Heart Association. *Circulation*. 2017;135:e50-e87.

6. Alliance for Innovation on Maternal Health (AIM). Cardiac conditions in obstetrical care. https://safehealthcareforeverywoman.org/aim/patient-safety-bundles/maternal-safety-bundles/cardiac-conditions-in-obstetrical-care/. Accessed April 2022.

16

Opioid Use Disorders

Merry I. Colella, MD
Yunping Li, MD

BACKGROUND

Substance use in pregnancy has escalated in recent years. Opioid-dependent patients frequently have severe postoperative pain due to opioid-induced hyperalgesia or tolerance.[1] Chronic use of either buprenorphine or methadone can result in these states.

Currently, due to lack of robust data and guidelines at a national level, healthcare providers have limited options for optimizing the management of this group of patients.

Coordinated care between obstetrics, anesthesia, addiction medicine, pediatrics, and social work aims to facilitate team collaboration and provide multimodal analgesia in order to provide the best possible postoperative pain control and patient satisfaction, improving maternal and neonatal outcomes.[2] This chapter will focus on the role of anesthesiologists in care of parturients with opioid use disorders (OUD) undergoing cesarean delivery. Given the unique needs of pregnant women with OUD, the anesthetic plan will need to be tailored to the patient's particular situation.

MEDICATION-ASSISTED TREATMENT (MAT) (TABLE 16-1)

- Pharmacokinetic and physiologic changes in pregnancy may require dose adjustments (usually increase), especially in the third trimester.
- The availability of buprenorphine for patients with OUD is the most significant event in addiction medicine since the introduction of methadone maintenance in the 1960s. Buprenorphine is the only opioid agonist currently approved for the treatment of OUD by a prescription in an office-based setting unlike methadone that must be managed in a licensed opioid treatment program.
- The human mu opioid receptor occupancy by buprenorphine is dose-related: 27% to 47% at 2 mg and 89% to 98% at 32 mg.[3]

TABLE 16-1 • Medication-Assisted Treatment for Opioid Use Disorders		
Medications	**Mechanisms**	**Half-Life**
Methadone	Full agonist	8-59 hours
Buprenorphine (Subutex)	Partial agonist	24-60 hours
Buprenorphine + naloxone (Suboxone)	Agonist and antagonist	~37 hours
Naltrexone	Pure opioid antagonist	13-14 hours
Buprenorphine extended release (Sublocade)	Partial agonist	43-60 days

- Naloxone is not orally active. It is used to reduce diversion because Suboxone causes severe withdrawal symptoms when injected.[4]
- Extended-release injectable buprenorphine (Sublocade) is given as a depot injection every 3 months to patients on a stable regiment of buprenorphine of at least 8 mg/day.[5]
- Opiate agonist/antagonist medications such as nalbuphine, butorphanol, and pentazocine are **contraindicated** as acute withdrawal can be precipitated in the opioid-dependent patient.

CLINICAL PRACTICE

Preoperative

- Continue buprenorphine-based or methadone MAT medications at the maintenance dose.
- If the patient is receiving methadone, she should not transition to partial agonist such as buprenorphine because of the significant risk of withdrawal.
- In patients taking naltrexone, taper to stop 72 hours prior to scheduled cesarean delivery.
- The patient should be scheduled for an obstetric anesthesia consult to allow for discussion of the patient's wishes and to provide reassurance and a plan for postpartum analgesia.

On the Day of Surgery

- The team will discuss the multimodal plan for pain control that tailors to individual patient.
- Neuraxial anesthesia is preferred when appropriate.
- Consider **NOT** using neuraxial morphine in a patient who is on
  - Methadone >80 mg/day or
  - Buprenorphine >8 mg/day or
  - Extended-release injectable buprenorphine.
- May consider using intrathecal (10 μg) or epidural (10 to 20 μg) dexmedetomidine (Chapter 6, "Dexmedetomidine").
- Consider low-dose intraoperative ketamine intravenously.
- Consider low thoracic epidural for postoperative analgesia.

Postoperative

- The obstetric anesthesia team manages the postoperative pain for the first 24 to 48 hours.
- Consulting chronic pain service may be considered.
- Continue the baseline dose of methadone or buprenorphine throughout the peripartum period.
- If the patient did not receive intrathecal morphine, use a hydromorphone or morphine patient-controlled analgesia for postoperative analgesia for breakthrough pain at 1.5 to 2 times higher dose than the routine dose, beginning in the recovery room. Parturients on methadone requires 70% more opioids following cesarean delivery.
- Administer scheduled, round-the-clock ketorolac and acetaminophen.
- For breakthrough pain, consider transversus abdominis plane or quadratus lumborum blocks or indwelling catheters.
- Alternatively, consider using low thoracic or high lumbar epidurals for continuous postoperative analgesia for the patient's breakthrough pain.
- May also use low-dose ketamine infusion at 0.1 to 0.3 mg/kg/h.
- Breastfeeding is beneficial in patients with OUD since it decreases the severity of symptoms from neonatal abstinence syndrome.

References

1. Jones HE, O'Grady K, Dahne J, et al. Management of acute postpartum pain in patients maintained on methadone or buprenorphine during pregnancy. *Am J Drug Alcohol Abuse*. 2009;35:151-156.

2. Leighton BL, Crock LW. Case series of successful postoperative pain management in buprenorphine maintenance therapy patients. *Anesth Analg*. 2017;125(5):1779-1783.

3. Greenwald M, Johanson CE, Bueller J, et al. Buprenorphine duration of action: mu-opioid receptor availability and pharmacokinetic and behavioral indices. *Biol Psych*. 2007;61:101-110.

4. The American College of Obstetrics and Gynecologists. Opioid use and opioid use disorder in pregnancy. Committee Opinion Number 711. *Obstet Gynecol*. 2017;130:e81-e94. https://www.acog.org/clinical/clinical-guidance/committee-opinion/articles/2017/08/opioid-use-and-opioid-use-disorder-in-pregnancy. Accessed April 2022.

5. Ling W, Shoptaw S, Goodman-Meza D. Depot buprenorphine injection in the management of opioid use disorder: from development to implementation. *Subst Abuse Rehabil*. 2019;10:69-78.

17

Neuraxial Anesthesia in Parturients on Anticoagulation

Merry I. Colella, MD

BACKGROUND

- Anticoagulation is a vital intervention to prevent venous thromboembolism and related maternal morbidity and mortality.
- The use of anticoagulation in parturients is becoming increasingly more common and has a substantial impact on the use and timing of neuraxial anesthetic procedures.
- As of yet, no professional society has published firm guidelines that adequately address the increased risk of epidural hematoma in anticoagulated obstetric patients. The American Society of Regional Anesthesia and Pain Medicine (ASRA) guidelines minimally differentiate between pregnant and nonpregnant patients and so do not account for the hypercoagulable state of pregnancy.[1]
- In a recent systematic review, an analysis of 52 parturients whose anticoagulation was not held for the recommended period prior to a neuraxial procedure did not find a single documented incidence of spinal epidural hematoma.[2]
- Using ASRA guidelines in an obstetric population would likely result in an inappropriate number of parturients being denied or delayed for neuraxial anesthesia, which leads to greater complications in those patients from the use of general anesthesia.
- The following guideline for parturients on unfractionated heparin (UFH) regimens is based on both a consensus statement from the Society for Obstetric Anesthesia and Perinatology,[3] related ASRA guidelines, and the experience of our senior staff.
- Establishing good communication with the patient, the obstetric team, and the nursing staff during both the antepartum period and upon the patient's arrival to the labor and delivery unit is essential and will aid in the adequate delivery of appropriate anesthetic care for labor analgesia in this patient population.

ANTEPARTUM

- Every patient on anticoagulation should receive an obstetric anesthesia consult appointment to discuss anesthetic options and the appropriate timing of neuraxial interventions in the setting of anticoagulation.

- We recommend all patients on low-molecular-weight heparin, such as enoxaparin, transition to UFH at 36 weeks, when possible. This allows for a more liberal timetable for neuraxial anesthesia should labor commence prior to the patient's due date.

Patients are advised not to administer any scheduled dose of UFH prior to arrival at the hospital if they are concerned that they may be going into labor.

PRIOR TO DELIVERY

Assess the patient's anticoagulation regimen, renal function, and bleeding history, and proceed as shown in Fig. 17-1.

OTHER CONSIDERATIONS

- For patients on enoxaparin, adhere to the ASRA guidelines for the timing of neuraxial as there is insufficient data currently to change this practice.
- For patients on heparin for >4 days, a platelet count should be performed within the past 24 hours prior to neuraxial procedures due to the risk of heparin-induced thrombocytopenia.

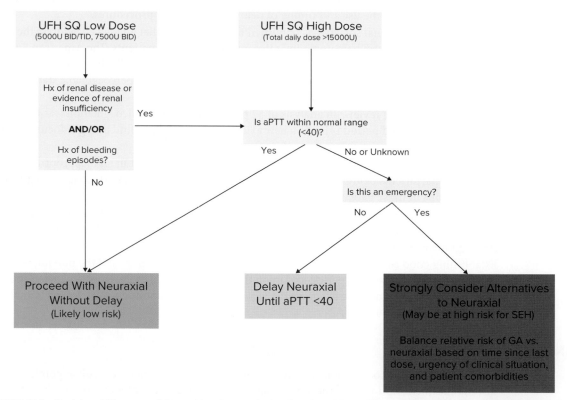

FIGURE 17-1 • Decision aid for neuraxial procedure in parturients on anticogulants. aPTT, activated partial thromboplastin time; GA, general anesthesia; Hx, history; SEH, subarachnoid or epidural hematoma; SQ, subcutaneous; UFH, unfractionated heparin.

References

1. Horlocker T, Vandermeuelen E, Kopp S, et al. Regional anesthesia in the patient receiving antithrombotic or thrombolytic therapy. American Society of Regional Anesthesia and Pain Medicine Evidence-Based Guidelines. 4th ed. *Reg Anesth Pain Med.* 2018;43:263-309.

2. Leffert L, Dubois H, Butwick A, et al. Neuraxial anesthesia in obstetric patients receiving thromboprophylaxis with unfractionated or low-molecular-weight heparin: a systematic review of spinal epidural hematoma. *Anesth Analg.* 2017;125(1):223-231.

3. Leffert L, Butwick A, Carvalho B, et al. The Society for Obstetric Anesthesia and Perinatology consensus statement on the anesthetic management of pregnant and postpartum women receiving thromboprophylaxis or higher dose anticoagulants. *Anesth Analg.* 2018;126(3):928-944.

18

Acute Management of Supraventricular Tachycardia

Maria C. Borrelli, DO
Jordan B. Strom, MD, MSc

BACKGROUND

Pregnancy is associated with increased arrythmia burden, and parturients with a history of arrythmia are at significant recurrence risk.[1]

Supraventricular tachycardia (SVT) includes a range of tachyarrythmias originating from a circuit or focus involving the atria or the atrioventricular node.[2,3] It manifests as a narrow complex (QRS < 120 ms), regular tachycardia.

PRESENTATION

Symptoms may include palpitations, lightheadedness, dizziness, syncope, dyspnea, and chest pain. May have abrupt onset (with or without abrupt termination). Prompt and correct diagnosis of SVT is necessary for efficient treatment. (See Table 18-1.)

MANAGEMENT (FIG. 18-1)

Assess hemodynamic status; stable or unstable?

- Telemetry (pulse audible).
- Blood pressure (repeated every 3 minutes).
- Pulse oximeter, may require supplemental oxygen and/or endotracheal intubation (if unstable).

TABLE 18-1 • Differentiating SVT from Sinus Tachycardia	
SVT	**Sinus Tachycardia**
Acute onset, acute cessation, often triggered by a premature atrial or ventricular (less common) beat[2]	Slow onset with progression to end
Typically stays at same rate Rate is usually 150-220 beats/min	Rate fluctuations Rate is usually 100-150 beats/min
Narrow QRS (most types) P waves may be subtle, hidden within the ST-segment, inverted, or bizarre morphologies[2,3]	Narrow QRS P waves present, upright in leads II, III, and aVF, and preceding the QRS complex

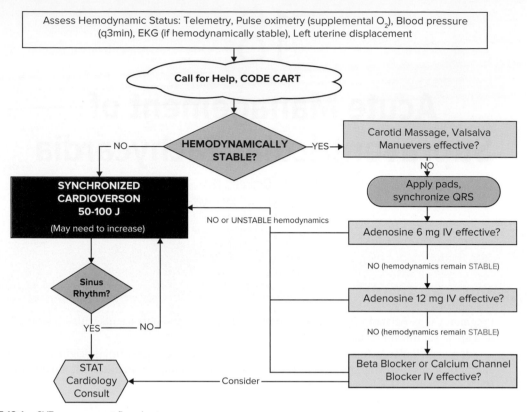

FIGURE 18-1 • SVT management flowchart.

- ○ Left uterine displacement.
- ○ 12-lead EKG (if hemodynamically stable).
- ○ Establish intravenous access.
- • Treatment[1]:
  - ○ Call for help, **CODE CART** nearby with pads.
  - ○ **Vagal manuevers** recommended first-line treatment for hemodynamically stable SVT[4,5]:
    - ▪ Valsalva (hold for 10 to 30 seconds; may be limited by patient participation).[6,7]
    - ▪ Carotid sinus pressure (auscultate for bruit prior; make sure to press high enough on neck) → manual pressure for 5 to 10 seconds.[6,7]
  - ○ **Adenosine** recommended first-line pharmacologic treatment for hemodynamically stable SVT[5,8]:
    - ▪ Make sure pads are placed prior to medication administration (pauses can cause arryth-mias, need to be ready for emergent cardioversion/defibrillation).
    - ▪ Synchronize to QRS complex (ensure NOT synchronized to T-wave).
    - ▪ Press "Print" button on cardioverter/defibrillator.
    - ▪ Administer **adenosine 6 mg intravenously (IV)** (half-life ~10 seconds) with rapid normal saline flush then lift arm immediately after administration to centrally distribute. If no effect, administer **adenosine 12 mg IV** in similar fashion.[4,8]
    - ▪ Common side effects include transient flushing, chest pain.[4]

- **Beta-blockers** recommended when adenosine is ineffective or contraindicated, and patient remains hemodynamically stable[5,8]:
  - Slow infusion is less likely to cause hypotension.[4,5,9]
  - **Metoprolol: 2.5 to 5 mg IV** over 2 minutes; may repeat in 10 minutes (up to 3 doses)[4] OR
  - **Propanolol: 1 mg IV** over 1 minute; may repeat 1 mg every 2 minutes (up to 3 doses).[4]
- **Calcium channel blockers** are reasonable for acute treatment when adenosine and beta-blockers are ineffective or contraindicated[5]:
  - Increased risk of hypotension and/or tocolysis.
  - **Verapamil: 5 to 10 mg IV** (0.075 to 0.15 mg/kg) over 2 minutes; may give an additional 10 mg (0.15 mg/kg) 30 minutes after first dose, then initiate a 0.005 mg/kg/min continuous IV infusion,[4] OR
  - **Diltiazem: 0.25 mg/kg IV** over 2 minutes; may start infusion at 5 to 10 mg/h (up to 15 mg/h).[4]
- **Synchronized cardioversion** is recommended if hemodynamically unstable or pharmacologic treatment is ineffective[5,10]:
  - Place pads such that the energy source and trajectory are directed away from uterus.[11]
  - Synchronize to QRS complex.
  - Press "Print" button on cardioverter/defibrillator.
  - Ensure left uterine displacement and no staff is touching the patient.
  - Energy dosing for parturient should be the same as in nonpregnant patients.[5]
  - Administer **50 to 100 J** biphasic energy.[8,10] If ineffective, may need to increase to 150 J.
- Post-cardioversion care:
  - Obtain cardiology consultation for IV/PO antiarrhythmic regimen.[10]
  - Fetal heart monitoring immediately post-cardioversion is recommended.[11]

References

1. Tamirisa KP, Elkayam U, Briller JE. Arrhythmias in pregnancy. *JACC Clin Electrophysiol.* 2022;8(1):120-135.
2. Kotadia ID, Williams SE, O'Neill M. Supraventricular tachycardia: an overview of diagnosis and management. *Clin Med (Lond).* 2020;20:43-47.
3. Ganz LI, Friedman PL. Supraventricular tachycardia. *N Engl J Med.* 1995;332:162-173.
4. Page RL, Joglar JA, Caldwell MA, et al. 2015 ACC/AHA/HRS Guideline for the management of adult patients with supraventricular tachycardia. *Circulation.* 2016;133(14):e506-e574. www.ahajournals.org.
5. Ghosh N, Luk A, Derzko C, et al. The acute treatment of maternal supraventricular tachycardias during pregnancy: a review of the literature. *J Obstet Gynaecol Can.* 2011;33:17-23.
6. Lim SH, Anantharaman V, Teo WS, et al. Comparison of treatment of supraventricular tachycardia by Valsalva maneuver and carotid sinus massage. *Ann Emerg Med.* 1998;31:30-35.
7. Waxman MB, Wald RW, Sharma AD, et al. Vagal techniques for termination of paroxysmal supraventricular tachycardia. *Am J Cardiol.* 1980;46:655-664.
8. Blomstrom-Lundqvist C, Scheinman MM, Alio EM, et al. ACC/AHA/ESC guidelines for the management of patients with supraventricular arrhythmias—executive summary. *J Am Coll Cardiol.* 2003;42:1493-1531.
9. Qasqas SA, McPherson C, Frishman WH, et al. Cardiovascular pharmacotherapeutic considerations during pregnancy and lactation. *Cardiol Rev.* 2004;12:201-221.
10. Adult Tachycardia with a Pulse Algorithm. American Heart Association Guidelines 2020. cpr.heart.org. Accessed March 2022.
11. Tromp CHN, Nanne ACM, Pernet PJM, et al. Electrical cardioversion during pregnancy: safe or not? *Neth Heart J.* 2011;19:134-136.

19

Thrombocytopenia

Philip E. Hess, MD

DEFINITION OF THROMBOCYTOPENIA

Platelet counts (PC) less than 150,000/mm³ are defined as thrombocytopenia. Mean PC decrease in all pregnant women, beginning in the first trimester.[1] Gestational thrombocytopenia is a diagnosis of exclusion in a healthy woman with uncomplicated pregnancy. PC may decrease further in a woman with pregnancy-related complications or preexisting thrombocytopenia.

ETIOLOGY OF THROMBOCYTOPENIA

- Gestational thrombocytopenia: affects 7% to 11% of pregnant women.[2] Usually, it is mild and stable when platelet count is near or above 100,000/mm³.
- Preeclampsia: accounts for 5% to 21% of cases of thrombocytopenia. Platelet function may be impaired. A **severe feature** of preeclampsia is hemolysis, elevated liver enzymes, and low platelet count (HELLP) syndrome.
- Acute placental abruption.
- Acute fatty liver of pregnancy.
- Idiopathic thrombocytopenic purpura (ITP).
- Disseminated intravascular coagulation.
- Thrombotic thrombocytopenic purpura and hemolytic-uremic syndrome, due to congenital or acquired ADAMTS13 (A Disintegrin-like Metalloprotease domain with ThromboSpondin type 1 motifs) deficiency.
- Drug-induced thrombocytopenia (e.g., heparin).

IMPACT ON FETUS AND NEONATES

- Gestational thrombocytopenia: poses no risk to the fetus.
- ITP: there is a 10% to 25% risk of fetal thrombocytopenia.
- Preeclampsia: increases risk (2%) of thrombocytopenia in neonates.

THROMBOCYTOPENIA AND SAFETY OF NEURAXIAL ANESTHESIA

A routine PC is not necessary in the healthy parturients before neuraxial procedures.[3]

However, a lack of high-quality data surrounds the safe placement of a neuraxial catheter in the parturients with thrombocytopenia. The threshold may vary in different providers and different patients and different thrombocytopenic disorders. The first society consensus statement

TABLE 19-1 • Suggested Interval Between the Time of Platelet Count and the Time of Neuraxial Placement	
Clinical Scenarios	**Intervals**
Preeclampsia	Within 24 hours
Preeclampsia with severe features	Within 12 hours
Any case with unstable platelet count	Within 4 hours
Acute placental abruption	Within 2-4 hours

on neuraxial procedures in obstetric patients was published in 2021, providing the best available evidence and clinical decision aid in the setting of thrombocytopenia.[4]

- Neuraxial anesthesia is considered safe when PC is ≥**70,000/mm³** in obstetric patients with gestational thrombocytopenia, ITP, and hypertensive disorders of pregnancy, and PC is stable, function is normal, and patient is not taking antiplatelet or anticoagulant drugs.
- Recommend using flexible catheter.
- Recheck PC before removal of an epidural catheter.
- Consider thromboelastography when PC is between 60,000 and 70,000/mm³.
- When PC is trending down, the interval between the time of PC and neuraxial placement should be taken into consideration. Highly recommend an early epidural placement to the patient before PC decreases further.
- Our practice recommendations are listed in Table 19-1.

References

1. Reese JA, Peck JD, Deschamps DR, et al. Platelet counts during pregnancy. *N Engl J Med*. 2018;379:32-43.
2. ACOG Practice Bulletin Number 207. Thrombocytopenia in pregnancy. *Obst Gynecol*. 2019;133:e181-e193.
3. Practice Guidelines for Obstetric Anesthesia: An updated report by the American Society of Anesthesiologists Task Force on Obstetric Anesthesia and the Society for Obstetric Anesthesia and Perinatology. *Anesthesiology*. 2016;124(2):270-300.
4. Bauer ME, Arendt K, Beilin Y, et al. The Society for Obstetric Anesthesia and Perinatology interdisciplinary consensus statement on neuraxial procedures in obstetric patients with thrombocytopenia. *Anesth Analg*. 2021;132(6):1531-1544.

20

Nonobstetric Surgery During Pregnancy

John J. Kowalczyk, MD

BACKGROUND

Nonobstetric surgery during pregnancy is common and occurs in between 0.3% and 2.2% of pregnancies. Retrospective human studies have not conclusively shown that any anesthetic agent results in increased congenital abnormalities. The conclusions of past studies have suggested possible teratogenic effects associated with nitrous oxide and benzodiazepines. However, more recent large retrospective studies have not supported these findings. General timing principles include[1]:

- If surgery is elective, defer until postpartum if appropriate.
- If surgery is nonelective and can be delayed without maternal harm, postpone until the second trimester (first trimester—potential teratogenic risk; third trimester—preterm labor risk).
- If surgery is urgent or emergent, proceed as necessary.

When a decision for surgery has been made, it is essential to begin planning and coordination. Early communication with obstetricians is important to ensure appropriate pre-, post-, and possible intraoperative fetal heart rate (FHR) monitoring is available. Prior to 22 to 24 weeks, only pre- and postoperative FHR monitoring is typically performed. Intraoperative monitoring is typically reserved for after the age of viability (>24 weeks) and may not be performed based on obstetrician and patient discretion. If intraoperative monitoring is performed, additional resources must be in place to allow for urgent or emergent cesarean delivery.

Necessary additional resources include:

- A labor and delivery nurse in the operating room (OR) to monitor the FHR and an obstetrician be available on standby to interpret the FHR and perform cesarean delivery.
- A cesarean delivery surgical tray needs to be in the OR at the start of the case along with neonatal resuscitation equipment, including a neonatal warmer.
- A 30-degree hip wedge should be available for left uterine displacement (LUD).
- Obstetricians may want to dose perioperative glucocorticoids for infant lung maturity (requires 48 hours for full effect).

PREOPERATIVE

- Perform evaluation, consent, and discuss plan with obstetrician and surgery team.
- Administer sodium citrate 30 mL orally <30 minutes before induction, if >12 to 16 weeks of gestational age.
  - May consider metoclopramide 10 mg and/or ranitidine 30 mg IV, >30 minutes prior to induction.
- Midazolam is not contraindicated; utilize it if necessary.

INTRAOPERATIVE

- Goal is to maintain appropriate pregnancy homeostasis.
- Pregnancy has been shown to be associated with increased sensitivity to sedatives, anesthetics, opioids, and local anesthetics.
- Maintain normotension.
- If the patient is greater than 20 weeks gestation (uterus at or above the umbilicus), it is crucial to place the patient in LUD prior to induction.
- Recommended initial ventilator settings of 6 to 8 mL/kg of ideal body weight and a respiratory rate of 14 to 18/min.
  - There is a *respiratory alkalosis* in pregnancy with a normal $PaCO_2$ of 30 mm Hg. The ventilator setting should be titrated to maintain this $PaCO_2$ near baseline.
- Volatile anesthetic minimum alveolar concentration (MAC) decreased by 20% to 30% in pregnancy.
- It is essential to be aware that volatile anesthetics and fentanyl may cause decreased variability of FHR (variability is not typically seen until >25 to 27 weeks).
- Volatile anesthetics cause dose-dependent uterine relaxation. If uterine contractions are noted by the obstetric team, consider increasing MAC or administer tocolytics in consultation with the obstetric attending (nitroglycerin 50 to 200 µg IV or terbutaline 0.25 mg IM).
- For laparoscopic surgery, maintain a low peritoneum insufflation pressure (<15 mm Hg).
- Avoid nonsteroidal anti-inflammatory drugs (NSAIDs) in the third trimester due to the risk of premature closure of ductus arteriosus.
- Safe to use opioids.
- Dexmedetomidine crosses the placenta and may cause fetal bradycardia at high dose, use with caution.
- For reversal of neuromuscular blockade:
  - Be aware that neostigmine crosses the uteroplacental barrier to a greater degree than glycopyrrolate. The use of glycopyrrolate with neostigmine may lead to marked fetal bradycardia, which may prompt obstetricians to initiate emergent cesarean.
  - Atropine will cross the uteroplacental barrier and may be used as an adjunct for reversal. This may cause both maternal and fetal tachycardia.
  - The data on the use of sugammadex is limited at this time. Studies show that sugammadex binds steroid hormones, such as progesterone, and eliminate them. Since progesterone is critical to the maintenance of pregnancy, the current expert opinion does not recommend its use in patients in early pregnancy. For patients at term or near-term pregnancy, the task force recommends judicious use due to unknown effects on lactation (Society for Obstetric Anesthesia and Peritonatology Statement on Sugammadex 2019).

- Pay careful attention to extubation with the patient maintaining appropriate respiratory physiology, fully awake and following commands.
  - Consider the placement of an oral gastric tube to empty the gastric contents if the patient did not meet NPO guidelines or there is a concern for a full stomach.
  - The majority of respiratory-related deaths occurred during emergence, extubation, and recovery.[2,3]

POSTOPERATIVE

- Avoid NSAIDs in the first and third trimesters.
- Evaluate for typical postoperative issues, including pain and nausea/vomiting.
- The patient may need transport to the recovery room in the labor and delivery. Obstetricians will likely obtain postoperative FHR tracing and monitor for contractions.
- Venous thrombosis prophylaxis should be considered if the patient is expected to be admitted.

References

1. ACOG Committee Opinion No. 474: Nonobstetric surgery during pregnancy. ACOG Committee on Obstetric Practice. *Obstet Gynecol*. 2011;117(2 Pt 1):420-421.
2. Mhyre JM. A series of anesthesia-related maternal deaths in Michigan, 1985-2003. *Anesthesiology*. 2007;106(6):1096-1104.
3. Kodali BS, Chandrasekhar S, Bulich LN, et al. Airway changes during labor and delivery. *Anesthesiology*. 2008;108(3):357-362.

21

Trial of Labor After Cesarean

Mohammed Idris, MD

BACKGROUND

Cesarean delivery (CD) is the most frequently performed surgery in the United States, and the rates have increased since the early 1970s.[1] Up to 30% of these are repeat CDs. The American College of Obstetricians and Gynecologists (ACOG) released a statement that "in the absence of a contraindication, a woman with one previous CD with a lower uterine segment incision should be counseled and encouraged to undergo a trial of labor."

PREANESTHETIC EVALUATION

Trial of labor after cesarean (TOLAC) has progressively become more commonplace throughout the United States. Despite this, risks associated with TOLAC require a higher level of care and additional considerations (Table 21-1). This includes:

- A multidisciplinary team including obstetricians, nursing, blood bank, neonatologists, and a dedicated in-house anesthesiologist
- Large-bore IV (18-16G)
- NPO (nothing by mouth) except clear liquids once in active labor
- Type and screen or type and crossmatch
- Early recognition of comorbidities
- Early epidural placement for TOLAC—this has been shown to increase patient acceptance rate of TOLAC

TABLE 21-1 • Benefits of Planned Vaginal Birth After Cesarean and Planned Repeat Cesarean Delivery

Benefits of VBAC	Benefits of Elective Repeat CD
• Less chance of placenta accreta spectrum in subsequent pregnancies • Less postoperative pain, early mobilization, shorter length of stay in hospital • Lower respiratory morbidity in newborn • Surgical risks associated with CD are not present • Less maternal morbidity	• Less chance of obstetric hemorrhage, blood transfusion, emergency hysterectomy as seen with uterine rupture • Lower perinatal morbidity and mortality like hypoxic encephalopathy, brachial plexus injury • Perinatal mortality not increased even if delivered after 39 weeks

CD, cesarean delivery; VBAC, vaginal birth after cesarean.

TABLE 21-2 • Prediction of Successful Vaginal Birth After Cesarean	
Factors Favoring Successful VBAC	**Factors Not In Favor Of Successful VBAC**
• Previous VBAC or vaginal delivery • One previous CD • Spontaneous labor	• No prior vaginal delivery • More than one prior CD • CD for dystocia, cephalopelvic disproportion or failed induction • Induction/augmentation of labor • Maternal obesity body mass index >40 kg/m² • Fetal macrosomia (>4000 g) • Gestational age >41 weeks • Coexisting conditions including oligo/polyhydramnios, chorioamnionitis • Black or Hispanic race/ethnicity

CD, cesarean delivery; VBAC, vaginal birth after cesarean.

- Constant communication with obstetricians regarding the progress of labor
- Availability of an operating room for emergency CD
- TOLAC in twin pregnancy: successful in about 45% to 70% of parturients with uterine rupture rate at about 0.9%

Vaginal birth after cesarean (VBAC) risk score for successful TOLAC can easily be estimated with an online calculator (Table 21-2).[2]

CONTRAINDICATIONS TO TOLAC

- Previous transmural or large myomectomy
- Classic uterine scar
- History of uterine rupture
- Placenta previa
- Placenta accreta spectrum
- Untreated genital herpes simplex virus infection
- Untreated human immunodeficiency virus infection

LABOR NEURAXIAL ANALGESIA

Labor analgesia is **NOT** contraindicated in TOLAC patients. Low concentration epidural analgesia does not mask signs of rupture, does not decrease success rates of VBAC, and improves acceptance rates of TOLAC.[3,4] Moreover, existing epidural will decrease the incidence of general anesthesia in the case of emergent cesarean if needed (Chapter 38, "Neuraxial Labor Analgesia").

UTERINE RUPTURE

Incidence

Rare but serious complications can result in perinatal death and long-term disability. The incidence is about 0.02% for elective repeat CD, 0.5% for VBAC after one previous CD, and 1.6% for VBAC after two previous CD.[5]

Risks Factors for Uterine Rupture[6,7]

- Induction of labor
- Advanced maternal age >40 years old
- Fetal macrosomia >4000 g
- Gestational age >40 weeks
- More than one prior CD
- Pregnancy interval <24 months
- Previous fundal or high vertical hysterotomy

Clinical Features of Uterine Rupture.[6] These are listed in Table 21-3.

Management of Uterine Rupture[9]

- Check maternal responsiveness
- Call for help
- Airway/Breathing:
  - High flow oxygen
  - Consider tracheal intubation if the patient cannot protect the airway or maintain oxygenation
- Circulation:
  - Maintain left uterine displacement
  - Obtain additional large-bore IV access, send laboratory tests (CBC, coagulation panel, fibrinogen, thromboelastography, lactate, venous blood gas)
  - Activate massive transfusion protocol
  - Fluid resuscitation with crystalloids and blood products
  - Consider tranexamic acid after fetal delivery
  - Immediate transfer to the operating room
  - Anesthesia options: epidural bolus if hemodynamically stable or general anesthesia if unstable
  - Arterial line for monitoring and blood sampling
  - Central venous line for vasopressors
  - Consider cell salvage
  - Maintain normothermia

TABLE 21-3 • Clinical Features of Uterine Rupture	
Fetal	**Maternal**
• Abnormal fetal heart rate pattern (most consistent sign) • Loss fetal station	• Acute abdominal pain: Persistent pain between contractions, increased epidural bolus requirements, scar tenderness • Nausea and vomiting, shortness of breath, diaphoresis (most likely due to free air or blood in the abdomen) • Vaginal bleeding • Increased uterine contraction or loss of uterine contraction • Maternal hemodynamic instability, increased lactate, increased metabolic acidosis • Frequent epidural dosing[8]

References

1. The American College of Obstetricians and Gynecologists (ACOG). Vaginal birth after cesarean delivery. *Obstet Gynecol.* 2019;133(2):e110-e127.

2. VBAC risk score for successful vaginal delivery (Flamm Model). https://www.mdcalc.com/vbac-risk-score-successful-vaginal-delivery-flamm-model. Accessed April 2022.

3. Grisaru-Granovsky S, Bas-Lando M, Drukker L, et al. Epidural analgesia at trial of labor after cesarean (TOLAC): a significant adjunct to successful vaginal birth after cesarean (VBAC). *J Perinat Med.* 2018;46(3):261-269.

4. Hawkins JL. The anesthesiologist's role during attempted VBAC. *Clin Obstet Gynecol.* 2012;55(4):1005-1013.

5. Holmgren CM. Uterine rupture associated with VBAC. *Clin Obstet Gynecol.* 2012;55(4):978-987.

6. Landon MB, Frey H. Uterine rupture: after previous cesarean birth. *UpToDate.* https://www.uptodate.com/contents/uterine-rupture-after-previous-cesarean-birth. Accessed April 2022.

7. Landon MB, Hauth JC, Leveno KJ, et al. Maternal and perinatal outcomes associated with a trial of labor after prior cesarean delivery. *N Engl J Med.* 2004;351:2581-2589.

8. Cahill AG, Odibo AO, Allsworth JE, Macones GA. Frequent epidural dosing as a marker for impending uterine rupture in patients who attempt vaginal birth after cesarean delivery. *Am J Obstet Gynecol.* 2010; 202:355.e1-355.e3555.

9. Plaat F, Shonfeld A. Major obstetric hemorrhage. *BJA Educ.* 2015;15(4):190-193.

22

Emerging Role of Ultrasound in Obstetric Patients

Aidan Sharkey, MD

INTRODUCTION

Point-of-care ultrasound (POCUS) encompasses an umbrella term for the use of ultrasound for diagnostic, monitoring, or therapeutic purposes. The evolution of ultrasound devices from large cart-based machines to handheld pocket probes has expanded the pool of users for this technology as well as its range of applications.[1] Obstetric anesthesiologists have a wide range of use for POCUS in both low- and high-risk parturients. The routine application of POCUS may encompass its use for facilitating procedures, such as vascular access, regional anesthesia techniques as well as assessing airway/lung/cardiac/intracranial and abdominal pathologies that may be encountered in the peripartum period (Fig. 22-1). The integration of POCUS into clinical practice was once deemed a desired skill but is fast becoming a prerequisite skill for obstetrical anesthesiologists to provide best patient care. This chapter will focus on the current and evolving use of ultrasound within obstetric anesthesia. Detailed description of ultrasound technology along with descriptive methods of obtaining and optimizing views is beyond the scope of this chapter.

CLINICAL APPLICATIONS

Neuraxial Procedures

Neuraxial anesthesia is the most common procedure performed by obstetric anesthesiologists and is traditionally performed using a landmark technique. Patient characteristics such as obesity, scoliosis, lordosis, and previous spine surgery along with pregnancy-related changes such as edema can sometimes make this procedure difficult and result in a higher incidence of complications such as inadvertent dural puncture and paresthesia. In patients with difficulty to palpate landmarks preprocedural ultrasound has been shown to reduce the number of attempts, improve the efficacy of neuraxial anesthesia, and result in improved patient satisfaction.[2]

Lung Ultrasound

Hypoxia due to pulmonary edema can often complicate pregnancy-related diseases such as preeclampsia or patients undergoing massive transfusion due to postpartum hemorrhage. Point-of-care lung ultrasound has proven itself to be both sensitive and specific in the diagnosis of pulmonary edema and can direct and monitor care in these patients. Lung ultrasound can also be

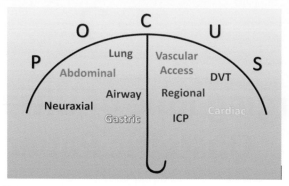

FIGURE 22-1 • Scope of POCUS used by obstetric anesthesiologists for diagnostic, monitoring, and procedural guidance purposes. DVT, deep vein thrombosis; ICP, intracranial pressure.

used to assess for pneumothorax in patients who may have had a central venous catheters placed for their peripartum care.

Airway Assessment

Difficult and failed intubations are more common in obstetric patients undergoing general anesthesia. Surgical airway access may be required for patients in whom the airway cannot be secured, and oxygenation is unable to be achieved. In this emergency situation, ultrasound identification of the cricothyroid membrane has been shown to be superior to digital palpation and may lead to a higher success rate if emergency cricothyroidotomy.[3]

Cardiac Ultrasound

Hemodynamic instability may occur for a multitude of reasons in the peripartum period. Acute right ventricular dysfunction due to pulmonary embolism (PE) or amniotic fluid embolism (AFE), hypovolemia due to acute hemorrhage, or left ventricular dysfunction due to postpartum cardiomyopathy all have similar presentations of a patient in an acute shocked state; however, the management will differ based on the acute pathology. Point-of-care cardiac ultrasound can be quickly used to help differentiate between the various causes of shock and direct therapeutic interventions more precisely.[4]

Cardiogenic shock due to postpartum cardiomyopathy can be diagnosed on transthoracic echocardiography (TTE) as left ventricular failure and is often accompanied by dilated chamber size (Fig. 22-2A). Obstructive shock due to acute PE or AFE will be seen on TTE as flattening of the interventricular septum in diastole and/or systole due to elevated right ventricular volume and/or pressure along with acute right ventricular dysfunction (Fig. 22-2B). Hypovolemic shock due to hemorrhage can be diagnosed with TTE by low left ventricular end systolic volume (kissing ventricle sign) (Fig. 22-2C). Fluid responsiveness can also be assessed by estimating inferior vena cava size and collapsibility. Correct interpretation as to the cause of shock can help guide treatment in these patients.

Gastric Ultrasound

Aspiration of gastric contents in patients undergoing general anesthesia (GA) for cesarean delivery or postpartum interventions carries significant morbidity. Real-time ultrasound assessment of gastric content is an easy and reliable method to evaluate gastric volumes prior to induction of GA. Multiple studies have documented good correlation between gastric antral cross-sectional

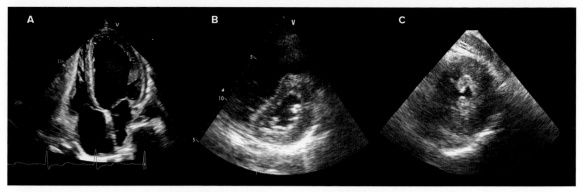

FIGURE 22-2 • Types of shock seen by obstetric anesthesiologists as visualized by echocardiography. **(A)** Dilated ventricle with low ejection fraction causing cardiogenic shock seen in postpartum cardiomyopathy. **(B)** RV dysfunction characterized by a dilated RV and flattening of the interventricular septum (D-shaped septum) seen in obstructive shock caused by pulmonary or amniotic fluid embolism. **(C)** Obliteration of left ventricular cavity (kissing ventricle sign) seen in hypovolemic shock caused by massive postpartum hemorrhage. RV, right ventricle.

area and predicted gastric volume. Using gastric ultrasound, it is possible to individually assess gastric aspiration risk and help plan airway management and the need for rapid sequence intubation.[5]

Abdominal Ultrasound

In patients with preeclampsia who present with epigastric pain, abdominal ultrasound can be used to detect liver subcapsular hematoma (Fig. 22-3A). Hepatic rupture should be suspected if free fluid is seen in the perihepatic space (Fig. 22-3B). Timely diagnosis and prompt intervention of these complications can decrease maternal morbidity and mortality. Abdominal ultrasound can also help to identify internal bleeding after cesarean delivery and retroperitoneal hematoma from extension of a cervical laceration in hemodynamically unstable patients.

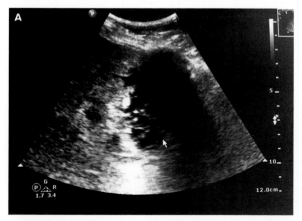
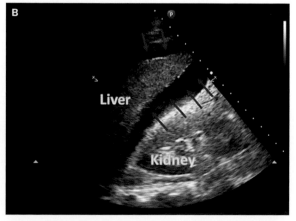

FIGURE 22-3 • **(A)** Subcapsular hematoma in a parturient with preeclampsia with severe features. **(B)** Free fluid (*red arrows*) in the perihepatic space indicating visceral bleeding in a patient with preeclampsia and a ruptured subscapular hematoma.

Intracranial Pressure

Raised intracranial pressure (ICP) in patients with preeclampsia can be seen in some patients as increased optic nerve diameter as measured with POCUS.[6] Further, assessing ICP ultrasound measurements of the optic nerve sheath may allow evaluation of cerebrospinal leak and thus supplement epidural blood patch.

Peripheral Nerve Blocks

Pain after cesarean delivery can have a significant impact on postoperative recovery and early infant bonding. The current gold standard for managing post-cesarean pain involves neuraxial opioid; however, not all patients may be suitable to receive this intervention. Ultrasound-guided transversus abdominis plane or quadratus lumborum nerve blocks offer a good alternative for these patients who cannot receive neuraxial opioids or who develop breakthrough pain.[7]

LIMITATIONS OF POCUS

POCUS has the potential to improve procedural success and safety while also diagnosing patient pathologies in a more accurate and timely fashion. However, we must also be cognizant of the limitations of POCUS. Access to and maintenance of equipment may present some physical barriers. Poor acoustic windows due to patient-related conditions can result in images that may be misintrepreted or are nondiagnostic. Finally, the current lack of training pathways and certification in POCUS results in inconsistent training standards between practitioners and institutions who utilize POCUS. Developing standards for training and maintaining competency is crucial if there is to be successful implementation of POCUS.

CONCLUSION

POCUS is an emerging technology that has multiple potential uses for the obstetric anesthesiologist to help diagnose and manage patients who encounter complications. Its use can also be incorporated into performed procedures to enhance safety and improve success of these procedures. This technology should be embraced by obstetric anesthesiologists to better care for our patients in the peripartum period.

References

1. Baribeau Y, Sharkey A, Chaudhary O, et al. Handheld point-of-care ultrasound probes: the new generation of pocus. *J Cardiothorac Vasc Anesth*. 2020;34(11):3139-3145.
2. Sahin T, Balaban O, Sahin L, et al. A randomized controlled trial of preinsertion ultrasound guidance for spinal anaesthesia in pregnancy: outcomes among obese and lean parturients: ultrasound for spinal anesthesia in pregnancy. *J Anesth*. 2014;28:413-419.
3. You-Ten KE, Siddiqui N, Teoh WH, Kristensen MS. Point-of-care ultrasound (POCUS) of the upper airway. *Can J Anaesth*. 2018 Apr;65(4):473-484.
4. Dennis AT, Stenson A. The use of transthoracic echocardiography in postpartum hypotension. *Anesth Analg*. 2012;115:1033-1037.
5. Perlas A, Arzola C, Van de Putte P. Point-of-care gastric ultrasound and aspiration risk assessment: a narrative review. *Can J Anaesth*. 2018;65(4):437-448.
6. Brzan Simenc G, Ambrozic J, Prokselj K, et al. Ocular ultrasonography for diagnosing increased intracranial pressure in patients with severe preeclampsia. *Int J Obstet Anesth*. 2018;36:49-55.
7. Chin KJ, McDonnell JG, Carvalho B, Sharkey A, Pawa A, Gadsden J. Essentials of our current understanding: abdominal wall blocks. *Reg Anesth Pain Med*. 2017;42(2):133-183.

23

Thromboelastography

John J. Kowalczyk, MD

BACKGROUND

Viscoelastic testing allows for the rapid assessment of the hemostatic properties of **whole blood**, measuring clot formation, strength, and breakdown.[1] The most common forms of viscoelastic testing commercially available include rotational thromboelastometry (ROTEM) and thromboelastography (TEG). These tests both evaluate hemostasis in a similar fashion and with a similar graphical result, although they contain slightly different proprietary terminology. TEG has traditionally been performed by combining whole blood with reagents in an oscillating cup with a suspended pin and associated torsion wire. The new TEG 6s is a cartridge-based system with four channels, piezoelectric actuator, and paired optical detection system.[2] This cartridge-based system improves ease of use and intradevice reliability.[3,4] Studies have shown that TEG/ROTEM can detect hypercoagulability of pregnancy, effects of heparin, patients at risk of thrombosis, and guide transfusion in postpartum hemorrhage.[5]

Postpartum hemorrhage (PPH) is the leading cause of maternal mortality worldwide and the leading cause of preventable death in the United States.[6] The rate of hemorrhage in the United States is 0.9% to 3.2%, and the rate of hemorrhage requiring transfusion is between 0.9% and 2.3%. Similar to transfusion in trauma, there has been an ongoing debate regarding the ideal ratio of blood product transfusion. Retrospective studies have shown a decrease in blood product usage, particularly fresh frozen plasma (FFP) and platelets, likelihood to be admitted to the intensive care unit, fewer hysterectomies, and shorter hospital length of stay in patients with severe PPH when the cases are managed with the use of viscoelastic testing.[7] Another study found the use of viscoelastic testing led to reduced blood product usage and rates of transfusion-associated complications.[8]

The inherent advantage of viscoelastic testing likely stems from the relative importance of fibrinogen in obstetric hemorrhage. Prior studies have shown that a fibrinogen level <200 mg/dL is the only value to have a 100% positive predictive value for PPH progressing to severe hemorrhage requiring transfusion.[9-11] A prior study has shown that fibrinogen measured by TEG is approximately 40 mg/dL greater than the traditional Clauss laboratory method.[12] These findings are consistent with our current study showing TEG 6s functional fibrinogen level (FLEV) approximately 45 mg/dL higher and returning a result more than 30 minutes faster.[13] Interestingly, recent work in TEG demonstrated that less than 15% of patients undergoing PPH had an increased rate of clot lysis.[14] This and other prior work potentially point to the underlying mechanism in most PPH complicated by medical bleeding due to underutilization of fibrinogen and hemodilution rather than clot lysis.

GOALS

- Identify coagulopathies that contribute to the progression of PPH (>1000 mL) to severe hemorrhage requiring transfusion.
- Rapidly assess the potential contribution of medical bleeding with a point-of-care test that allows quick, actionable results, often in less than 30 minutes.
- Manage hemorrhage with a goal-directed transfusion strategy that repletes the appropriate products while limiting exposure and complications from unneeded products.

CLINICAL PRACTICE

- TEG 6s is a cartridge-based system that allows for easy point-of-care utilization.
  - Remove a cartridge from the refrigerator and allow it to come to room temperature while completing the following steps.
- For TEG 6s global or lysis cartridges, blood should be collected in a blue top (citrate) vacutainer.
  - Cartridge choice:
    - For hemorrhage related to atony, we recommend the use of the Global TEG cartridge for faster results from K, Angle, and FLEV.
    - In the uncommon occurrence of hemorrhage related to amniotic fluid embolism (AFE) or disseminated intravascular coagulation (DIC), we recommend the use of the Lysis cartridge.
  - Ensure that the blue top is up to the fill line.
  - Allow the blood to incubate in the vacutainer for at least 10 minutes on its side.
- After powering up the system, follow the directions displayed on the screen, and when prompted, insert the cartridge and fill the cartridge chamber with blood to or slightly above the fill line.
- After a short time, the graph displays, allowing for interpretation while the test completes (Fig. 23-1).

INTERPRETATION AND BLOOD PRODUCT ADMINISTRATION

TEG 6s has been streamlined for interpretation. In doing so, TEG 6s attempts to separate the relative impact of platelets and fibrinogen with the creation of maximum amplitude (MA) in Citrated Rapid® TEG (CRT) and Citrated Functional Fibrinogen (CFF) channels. The key values are discussed below. Despite the discrete values, it has been our experience that significant derangements in any value may affect subsequent values. For example, very low R values will lead to changes in K, Angle, MA CRT, and MA CFF, and changes in K, Angle, or MA CFF will lead to a decrease in MA CRT.

Citrated Kaolin (CK) Reaction Time (R Time) (minutes)
- Definition: Clot time measured from the start of the test to initiation of the clot (2 mm).
- Decreased:
  - Enzymatic hypercoagulability.
  - Pregnant patients are naturally in a hypercoagulable state and will thus have a low-normal R time.

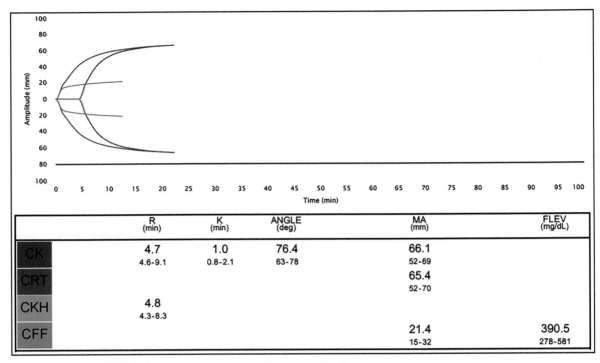

	R (min)	K (min)	ANGLE (deg)	MA (mm)	FLEV (mg/dL)
CK	4.7 4.6-9.1	1.0 0.8-2.1	76.4 63-78	66.1 52-69	
CRT				65.4 52-70	
CKH	4.8 4.3-8.3				
CFF				21.4 15-32	390.5 278-581

FIGURE 23-1 • Normal TEG 6s thromboelastogram results in a pregnant patient.

- Increased:
  - Enzymatic coagulopathy.
  - Etiology: Heparin activity (see the next section "CKH R Time"), dilutional coagulopathy, liver dysfunction secondary to preeclampsia with severe features or HELLP (hemolysis, elevated liver enzymes, low platelet count), congenital, or acquired factor deficiency.
  - Treatment: FFP or replacement of specific factors.

CK Heparinase (CKH) R Time (minute)

- Definition: Clot time measured from the start of the test to initiation of the clot (2 mm) in the presence of heparinase.
- Similar to CK R time (± 0.5 minute):
  - No or minimal residual heparin effect.
- Shorter than CK R time (>2 minute shorter):
  - Residual heparin or low-molecular-weight heparin effect.
  - Treatment: Heparin reversal, if in the setting of uncontrolled bleeding.

Kinetic (K) Time (minute)

- Definition: The speed of clot formation measured by the time it takes from clot initiation (2 mm) until the clot reaches a width of 20 mm.
- Increased:
  - Coagulopathy due to low fibrinogen.
  - Treatment and etiology: Refer to the section "MA CFF."

Alpha Angle (degrees)

- Definition: The speed of clot formation measured by the angle of a tangent line to the curve between the R and K from the horizontal line.
- Decreased:
  - Coagulopathy due to low fibrinogen.
  - Treatment and etiology: Refer to the section "MA CFF."
- Note: Alpha angle is inversely proportional to K time. By the nature of their respective definitions, as one increases, the other decreases and vice versa.

Maximum Amplitude (MA) (millimeter)

- Definition: Clot strength measured as the amplitude (mm) at the maximum curve width.
- Decreased:
  - Coagulopathy primarily due to low quantity or function of platelets.
  - Etiology and treatment: Refer to the section "MA CRT."
- Note: MA includes the contribution of fibrinogen; as such, management of patients with very low fibrinogen would also contribute to a decrease in MA, clouding the picture in management decisions. With TEG 6s, MA CRT and MA CFF were created to help limit confusion on management decisions.

MA CRT (millimeter)

- Definition: Clot strength is measured as the amplitude (mm) at the maximum curve width in the presence of kaolin and tissue factor. The addition of tissue factor allows immediate activation of both the intrinsic and extrinsic pathway skipping the R time and allowing for a more rapid result.
- Decreased:
  - Coagulopathy due to low platelets.
  - Etiology: Dilutional coagulopathy, platelet destruction due to HELLP syndrome, immune thrombocytopenic purpura, or thrombotic thrombocytopenic purpura.
  - Treatment: Platelets.
- Note: In the setting of decreased MA CRT and MA CFF, we would still recommend the replacement of fibrinogen first to correct for any spillover effect.

MA CFF (millimeter)

- Definition: Clot strength measured as the amplitude (mm) at the maximum curve width in the presence of kaolin, tissue factor, and a platelet inhibitor (abciximab). The addition of the platelet inhibitors allows for an isolated measurement of fibrinogen's contribution to clot strength.
- Decreased:
  - Coagulopathy due to low fibrinogen.
  - Etiology: Dilutional coagulopathy, AFE, DIC.
  - Treatment: Cryoprecipitate or fibrinogen concentrate.

Functional Fibrinogen Level (FLEV) (mg/dL)

- Definition: Clot strength as measured by MA CFF and then transformed into a more familiar function fibrinogen level.

- Decreased:
  - Coagulopathy due to low fibrinogen.
  - Etiology and treatment: Refer to the section "MA CFF."
- Note: Despite this value being presented in the same units as the traditional laboratory Clauss assay method, this is not a quantitative measurement of fibrinogen. Rather, it is a proprietary calculation of the "functional fibrinogen" level derived from MA CFF.

Lysis 30 (Lys30) (%)

- Definition: Clot lysis as expressed by the percentage decrease in amplitude at 30 minutes after MA compared to MA amplitude.
- Increased:
  - Coagulopathy due to lysis of the fibrin cross-bridge stabilizing the clot.
  - Etiology: AFE, DIC.
  - Treatment: Tranexamic acid.
- Note: As mentioned in the background, this does not appear to be present in the most common causes of obstetric hemorrhage—atony.

LIMITATIONS

Medications that cause selective platelet inhibition, such as aspirin and clopidogrel, will not be detected on a traditional TEG and must be evaluated by TEG Platelet Mapping.

References

1. Whiting D, DiNardo JA. TEG and ROTEM: technology and clinical applications. *Am J Hematol.* 2014;89(2):228-232.
2. Faraoni D, DiNardo J. Viscoelastic hemostatic assays: update on technology and clinical applications. *Am J Hematol.* 2021;96(10):1331-1337.
3. Gurbel PA, Bliden KP, Tantry US, et al. First report of the point-of-care TEG: a technical validation study of the TEG-6S system. *Platelets.* 2016;27:642-649.
4. Neal MD, Moore EE, Walsh M, et al. A comparison between the TEG 6s and TEG 5000 analyzers to assess coagulation in trauma patients. *J Trauma Acute Care Surg.* 2020;88:279-285.
5. Amgalan A, Allen T, Othman M, Ahmadzia HK. Systematic review of viscoelastic testing (TEG/ROTEM) in obstetrics and recommendations from the women's SSC of the ISTH. *J Thromb Haemost.* 2020;18(8):1813-1838.
6. Reale SC, Easter SR, Xu X, Bateman BT, Farber MK. Trends in postpartum hemorrhage in the United States from 2010 to 2014. *Anesth Analg.* 2020;130(5):e119-e122.
7. Snegovskikh D, Souza D, Walton Z, et al. Point-of-care viscoelastic testing improves the outcome of pregnancies complicated by severe postpartum hemorrhage. *J Clin Anesth.* 2018;44:50-56.
8. Mallaiah S, Barclay P, Harrod I, Chevannes C, Bhalla A. Introduction of an algorithm for ROTEM-guided fibrinogen concentrate administration in major obstetric haemorrhage. *Anaesthesia.* 2015;70(2):166-175.
9. Barclay P, Harrod I, Chevannes C, Bhalla A. Introduction of an algorithm for ROTEM-guided fibrinogen concentrate administration in major obstetric haemorrhage. *Anaesthesia.* 2015;70(2):166-175.
10. Charbit B, Mandelbrot L, Samain E, et al. The decrease of fibrinogen is an early predictor of the severity of postpartum hemorrhage. *J Thromb Haemost.* 2007;5(2):266-273.
11. Cortet M, Deneux-Tharaux C, Dupont C, et al. Association between fibrinogen level and severity of postpartum haemorrhage: secondary analysis of a prospective trial. *Br J Anaesth.* 2012;108(6):984-989.
12. Katz D, Hamburger J, Batt D, Zahn J, Beilin Y. Point-of-care fibrinogen testing in pregnancy. *Anesth Analg.* 2019;129(3):e86-e88.
13. Moldysz A, Borrelli M, Li Y, et al. Strong linear correlation between functional fibrinogen by thromboelastography 6S and fibrinogen level by Clauss method in pregnant women. Society for Obstetric Anesthesia and Perinatology 54th Annual Meeting. May 2022 Chicago, IL.
14. Arnolds DE, Scavone BM. Thromboelastographic assessment of fibrinolytic activity in postpartum hemorrhage: a retrospective single-center observational study. *Anesth Analg.* 2020;131(5):1373-1379.

24

Percutaneous Umbilical Blood Sampling

Sichao Xu, MD
Justin K. Stiles, MD

Percutaneous umbilical blood sampling (PUBS), or cordocentesis, is an ultrasound-guided intrauterine procedure to obtain access to the fetal circulation for diagnostic and potentially therapeutic interventions.

INDICATIONS OF PUBS

The most common indication for PUBS is to diagnose and treat severe fetal anemia.[1] Other indications include nonimmune hydrops and neonatal thrombocytopenia.

SPECIAL CONSIDERATIONS FOR PUBS

Bigelow and coauthors performed a single-center retrospective study which demonstrated that the average gestational age at the time of PUBS was 26.7 weeks, with 34.7% of cases performed before 24 weeks of gestation.[2]

Most centers use 20- or 22-gauge spinal needle under ultrasound guidance for access.

The most commonly accessed site is the umbilical vein at the placental cord insertion site. Other sites include the umbilical vein at the abdominal cord insertion site, free loop of the umbilical vein, intrahepatic vein, and the fetal heart.[1]

If intrauterine transfusion or a longer procedure time is expected, some centers use intravenous paralytics administered to the fetus to reduce fetal movement. Historically the use of pancuronium was more common; however, a double blinded study has found that atracurium (0.4 mg/kg) has less effect on fetal heart rate comparing to pancuronium (0.1 mg/kg).[3] Pancuronium is the drug of choice by the proceduralists at the authors' institution when muscle relaxant is needed. Rocuronium, one of the most widely used paralytics in the United States, has not been described in literature in PUBS.

RISKS AND COMPLICATIONS OF PUBS

- Bleeding from the puncture site (20% to 30%), usually self-limiting.[1]
- Fetal bradycardia (5% to 10%), usually resolves within 5 minutes.[1] This could be due to vasospasm of the umbilical artery, streaming of blood from the umbilical vein to the umbilical

artery, compression from a cord hematoma, etc.[4] Prolonged fetal bradycardia may necessitate emergent cesarean delivery or result in fetal loss.

- Incidence of pregnancy loss (within 2 weeks of procedure) varies. For fetuses without structural abnormalities or hydrops, the incidence is low (about 1%); for fetuses with hydrops especially nonimmune hydrops, the incidence is higher (10% to 30%).[1]

ANESTHETIC CONSIDERATIONS

Currently, there is no data regarding the preferred anesthesia technique for PUBS. The Society of Maternal-Fetal-Medicine recommends that when fetal viability is reached, PUBS should be performed near or within an operating room in case an emergent cesarean delivery (the incidence of which is rare and not well documented) is indicated.[1] Parturients over 24 weeks gestational age and who are pregnant with structurally abnormal fetuses may benefit from regional anesthesia. The anesthesiologists should assess patients on a case-by-case manner and be prepared for stat cesarean deliveries. If intrauterine transfusion and longer procedure time is anticipated, combined spinal and epidural anesthesia should be considered.

Ideal operating conditions include a comfortable, calm, and still patient. The procedure is not very stimulating. Prior to fetal viability, only local anesthetic infiltration is provided. Entry site will vary with gestational age and fetus/cord position. Nausea should be avoided as vomiting/retching could interfere with the delicate procedure. Early antiemetics, subhypnotic/anxiolytic propofol infusions, and left uterine displacement are encouraged. Minimize engaging the patient in conversation and encourage a steady breathing pattern during the needling portion of the procedure. If neuraxial anesthesia is used, an epidural catheter should be placed to prepare for prolonged procedures or conversion to emergent cesarean delivery. While neuraxial anesthesia is not essential, it could prevent the need for general anesthesia if an emergent cesarean is required.

References

1. Berry SM, Stone J, Berghella V. Fetal blood sampling. *Am J Obstet Gynecol*. 2013;209:170-180.
2. Bigelow CA, Cinelli CM, Little SE, Benson CB, Frates MC, Wilkins-Haug LE. Percutaneous umbilical blood sampling: current trends and outcomes. *Eur J Obstet Gynecol Reprod Biol*. 2016;200:98-101.
3. Mouw RJ, Klumper F, Hermans J, Brandenburg HC, Kanhai HH. Effect of atracurium or pancuronium on the anemic fetus during and directly after intravascular intrauterine transfusion: a double blind randomized study. *Acta Obstet Gynecol Scand*. 1999;78:763-767.
4. Peddi NC, Avanthika C, Vuppalapati S, Balasubramanian R, Kaur J, Chaithanya DN. A review of cordocentesis: percutaneous umbilical cord blood sampling. *Cureus*. 2021;13(7):e16423.

25

Ex Utero Intrapartum Treatment

Mohammed Idris, MD

Philip E. Hess, MD

BACKGROUND

Ex utero intrapartum treatment (EXIT) is a set of clinical procedures where a fetus with life-threatening airway or pulmonary abnormalities is partially delivered during cesarean section and is kept oxygenated through an attached placenta until treatment is completed. Fetal head and one or both shoulders are delivered for access during treatment; uterine relaxation during the treatment phase is paramount, as is preservation of uterine perfusion also is essential.

Principles of management of EXIT procedures are similar to that of nonobstetric surgeries in pregnancy, but with two surgical patients, mother and fetus. Fetal analgesia can be partially provided by maternal transfer of agents but also frequently requires intramuscular (IM) and intravenous (IV) administration of drugs.

Preparation for fetal resuscitation and maternal hemorrhage is important. With the ongoing controversy regarding the fetal neurotoxicity of anesthetic agents, minimizing the duration of exposure of the fetus to anesthetic agents is extremely important. The common indications and fetal physiologic consideration for EXIT procedures are listed in Table 25-1.

TABLE 25-1 · Fetal Considerations for EXIT Procedures	
Indications for EXIT	**Fetal Physiologic Parameters**
• Airway obstruction (cervical teratomas, cystic hygroma, lymphangiomas, micrognathia, intraoral masses)[1] • Congenital high airway obstruction syndrome, e.g., laryngeal atresia • Congenital goiter • Congenital diaphragmatic hernia • Mediastinal masses	• Fetal pain • Neuroendocrine response seen at 20 weeks • Thalamocortical connections seen at 24 weeks • Fetal cardiac output is proportional to heart rate • Lungs are fluid filled; 100 mL/day produced • Blood volume: 110-160 mL/kg • Coagulation factors are less functional • Minimal immune function

FIGURE 25-1 • Phases of EXIT procedure.

PHASES OF EXIT PROCEDURE (FIG. 25-1)

PREOPERATIVE PREPARATION (TABLE 25-2)[2,3]

- Assessment of maternal comorbidities
- Imaging studies for placental location, location of lesion, and fetal weight
- Ideal timing: Close to term, often 34 to 35 weeks of gestational age

TABLE 25-2• Anesthetic Considerations for EXIT Procedure	
Mother	**Fetus**
Two large bore IV (16G +18G)	Ultrasound with sterile cover
Arterial line under local anesthesia	Fentanyl (20 µg/kg), rocuronium (1-3 mg/kg) or vecuronium (0.2 mg/kg) and atropine (20 µg/kg) for intramuscular injection (IM)
Ephedrine and phenylephrine boluses and infusion	Emergency drugs: epinephrine (10 µg/kg), atropine (20 µg/kg)
Nitroglycerin boluses (50-100 µg) or infusion at 1 µg/kg/min if required	Pulse oximeter (with sterile sheath) dedicated for baby monitoring
Warm intravenous fluids	End-tidal CO_2 monitoring, gas analyzer
Sevoflurane or desflurane	Different size, styletted pediatric endotracheal tubes
Keep operating room warm	Sterile Ambu bag with manometer attached to oxygen source
Crossmatched blood	Foil for placement over fetal pulse oximeter probe to decrease ambient light interference
	Plastic bag to cover baby's head upon partial delivery
	24G catheter for IV access
	Crystalloid/blood (O negative, cytomegalovirus negative, leukocyte-reduced, irradiated, maternal crossmatched)
	Fetal/neonatal resuscitation cart

- Multidisciplinary meeting (anesthesiologists, obstetricians, pediatric surgeons, pediatric cardiologists, neonatologists, radiologists, nurse, blood bank).
- Maternal aspiration prophylaxis.
- IV lines for hemorrhage preparedness.
- Arterial line to assess fetal perfusion.
- General anesthesia with intubation is most often used.

INTRAOPERATIVE MANAGEMENT

- Lumbar epidural catheter may be considered after ruling out anticoagulation for intraoperative use and postoperative analgesia.
- Rapid sequence induction with propofol and succinylcholine.
- Left uterine displacement.
- Ultrasound exam of uterus and placenta to confirm placental location and fetal position.

Maintenance of Anesthesia

- Uterine relaxation with volatile agents up to 2 to 3 minimum alveolar concentration (MAC).
- Start phenylephrine infusion to maintain mean arterial pressure near normal.
- Repeat nitroglycerin boluses of 50 to 100 µg, if uterine activity is detected.
- The edge of uterine incision is clipped with special stapling device to minimize bleeding.
- 100% O_2 to mother till baby is delivered.
- Infuse warm fluids to the uterus to prevent uterine collapse and premature labor contractions.

Monitoring of Fetus

- Pulse oximeter on hand.
- Periodic cardiac ultrasound.
- Normal fetal pulse oximeter is between 40% and 70% (improves to 90% on ventilation of lungs).

Maintenance of Anesthesia for the Fetus

The medications include:

- Fentanyl (20 µg/kg)[1] IM
- Rocuronium (1 to 3 mg/kg) IM
- Vecuronium (0.2 mg/kg) IM
- Atropine (20 µg/kg) IM

Anesthesia After Delivery of Fetus

- Reduce volatile agents.
- Start total intravenous anesthesia (TIVA) and nitrous oxide.
- Start oxytocin (add additional uterotonics like methylergonovine, prostaglandins as required).

Management of Fetal Bradycardia (BOX 25-1)

BOX 25-1 • Fetal Bradycardia/Arrest Treatment

Causes:

- Umbilical cord compression/kinking/twisting
- Uterine contraction
- Placental abruption

Optimize mother:

- O_2 supplement
- Hemodynamics
- Left uterine displacement

Treatment:

- Epinephrine, atropine
- Reposition of fetus
- Chest compressions
- Fluid
- Blood transfusion

Complications

- Placental abruption, fetal bradycardia, blood transfusion, fetal death

Malignant Hyperthermia Patients

- Epidural analgesia has been reported.
- TIVA—Propofol with remifentanil and nitroglycerin infusion.
- Remifentanil crosses the placenta.

References

1. Butler CR, Maughan EF, Pandya P, Hewitt R. Ex utero intrapartum treatment (EXIT) for upper airway obstruction. *Curr Opin Otolaryngol Head Neck Surg.* 2017;25:119-126.

2. Dinges E, Heier J, Delgado C, Bollag L. Multimodal general anesthesia approach for ex utero intrapartum therapy (EXIT) procedures: two case reports. *Int J Obstet Anesth.* 2019;38:142-145.

3. Hirose S, Farmer DL, Lee H, et al. The ex utero intrapartum treatment procedure: looking back at the EXIT. *J Pediatr Surg.* 2004;39:375-380.

26

Cerclage

Yunping Li, MD
Scott A. Shainker, DO, MS

INTRODUCTION

Cervical insufficiency affects about 1% of all pregnancy. It is defined as painless cervical dilation in the second trimester. Cervical insufficiency can be preceded by cervical shortening (less than 2.5 cm). It is associated with an increased risk of preterm labor and birth.

The risks of cervical insufficiency include:

- Idiopathic
- Surgical trauma from loop electrosurgical excision procedures and cervical conization
- Repeated forced cervical dilation associated with dilation and curettage
- Obstetric lacerations
- Prior history of cervical insufficiency
- Congenital disorders: Mullerian duct abnormalities, Ehlers-Danlos syndrome, congenital deficiencies in collagen and elastin

TYPES OF CERCLAGES[1]

Transvaginal Cervical Cerclage

The McDonald and Shirodkar techniques are most often used. Both use nonabsorbable sutures and requite removal before the commencement of labor to avoid cervical trauma. In the McDonald procedure, a simple suture is placed in a "purse string" like manner circumferentially around the cervix; the Shirodkar procedure involves the dissection of the cervical mucosa in order to place the suture as close as possible to the internal OS of cervix. There is insufficient data to support the superiority of one surgical technique over another type.

Transabdominal Cervical Cerclage

It is accomplished through open laparotomy or laparoscopy. It can be performed during the late first trimester or the early second trimester or even in non-pregnant status. The stitch is placed at the internal OS and can be left in place between pregnancies. Cesarean delivery is the required mode of delivery subsequently. Transabdominal cervical cerclage is more invasive and is reserved for those who have failed vaginal cerclage.[2]

ANESTHETIC CONSIDERATIONS FOR CERCLAGES

In the patient with prior cervical insufficiency, or those with a history of preterm birth and a short cervix, cerclage is associated with significant reduction in preterm birth and the consequences of prematurity. Thus, the procedure itself can be urgent in nature; however, cerclage is contraindicated in the setting of painful contractions, bleeding, or uterine infection. Overall, cerclage is a very safe procedure with low risk of complications.

Although cerclage is an ambulatory procedure, the choice of anesthesia and dosing of spinal medication are most diversified. Here we will discuss the anesthetic considerations in general:

- Lithotomy position that may affect the spread of spinal block.
- Surgical duration varies, but it is usually less than 60 minutes.
- Intraoperative fetal monitoring is not used routinely as the procedure is always performed prior to fetal viability.
- Left uterine displacement if gestation age is greater than 18 weeks.
- Aggressively prevent and treat hypotension associated with regional anesthesia (Chapter 50, "Hypotension After Spinal Anesthesia").
- Regional anesthesia is preferred to minimize the fetal exposure to anesthetics and maternal risks related to general anesthesia.
- Sacral coverage is mandatory; so hyperbaric local anesthetics are desired. Spinal anesthesia with 1 to 1.2 mL of hyperbaric 0.75% bupivacaine (7.5 to 9 mg) is recommended. The patient should remain in the sitting position for 2 to 3 minutes after spinal to establish saddle block.
- In a recent randomized controlled trial,[3] 50 mg of intrathecal 3% chloroprocaine was compared to 9 mg of 0.75% hyperbaric bupivacaine both in combination with 15 µg of fentanyl for cervical cerclage; chloroprocaine provided similarly effective anesthesia and produced earlier resolution of motor block and shorter time to discharge. The authors emphasized that the chloroprocaine must be preservative free.
- 5% hyperbaric lidocaine is rarely used because of the risk of transient neurological symptoms.
- Use of intrathecal short-acting fentanyl (15 to 25 µg) is controversial. It can improve intraoperative analgesia and extend duration of blocks; however, the higher dose may contribute to postoperative urinary retention and delayed discharge.[4]
- Epidural anesthesia would be a poor choice as sacral sparing is common.
- In the setting of cervical dilation with exposed amniotic sac, maternal retching may result in deep Valsalva and increase the risk of rupture of the amniotic membranes; thus, adequate anesthesia and control of hypotension and vomiting is paramount.
- In the absence of hypotension, postoperative nausea and vomiting prophylaxis is not indicated for regional anesthesia.
- General anesthesia is an option if there are contraindications for regional anesthesia or patient's refusal.
- For transabdominal cerclage, general anesthesia is usually warranted.
- Postoperative pain is minimal. If needed, a short course (48 hours) of nonsteroidal anti-inflammatory drugs can be used; however, rarely it is needed. After discussion with the obstetrician, single dose of ketorolac is often considered safe.

References

1. The American College of Obstetrics and Gynecologists. Cerclage for the management of cervical insufficiency. Practice Bulletin Number 142, February 2014. Accessed May 2022.
2. Tushva OA, Cohen SL, McElrath TF, et al. Laparoscopic placement of cervical cerclage. *Rev Obstet Gynecol.* 2012;5:e158-e165.
3. Lee A, Shatil B, Landau R, et al. Intrathecal 2-chloroprocaine 3% versus hyperbaric bupivacaine 0.75% for cervical cerclage: a double-blind randomized controlled trial. *Anesth Analg.* 2022;134(3):624-632.
4. Hsu G, Li Y, Pratt SD. Optimal bupivacaine spinal for cervical cerclage: effect on ambulation, urination, PACU time and pain control. Society for Obstetric Anesthesia and Perinatology Annual Meeting 2013 San Juan, Puerto Rico.

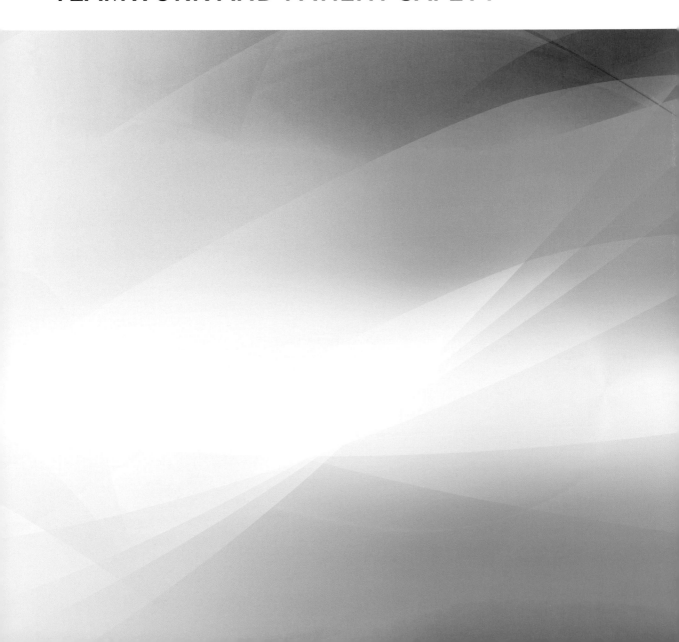

PART IV
TEAMWORK AND PATIENT SAFETY

27

Contingency Team

Josephine M. Hernandez, MD
Susan Craft, RN, MS
Janet C. Guarino, RN, MS

BACKGROUND

In 1999, the Institute of Medicine estimated that medical errors accounted for up to 98,000 deaths each year in the United States,[1] with the Joint Commission reporting that over 70% of adverse obstetric outcomes were due to failures in teamwork and communication.[2] In 2001, the Beth Israel Deaconess Medical Center (BIDMC) Department of Obstetrics and Gynecology teamed up with the Department of Defense and the Risk Management Foundation to develop a Crew Management Resource (CMR) team-based training curriculum in Obstetrics. The Labor and Delivery Unit was the first in obstetrics and one of the first in healthcare to apply CMR to clinical medicine. When BIDMC later reviewed its own Adverse Outcome Index (AOI) and Weighted Adverse Outcome Score (WAOS) data prior to this new CMR curriculum and training (from 1999 to 2001) and after CRM implementation (from 2003 to 2006), they found a 23% decrease in AOI and a 33.2% decrease in WAOS. That translates to 300 fewer women who experienced adverse events after CMR team training was implemented.[3]

One important prong of CRM team training is the creation of a Rapid Response Team, titled the **Contingency Team** at BIDMC, which is an organized team that is dedicated to responding to emergency obstetric situations, primarily STAT cesarean deliveries. The care of a parturient in distress may be compromised secondary to overcrowding and lack of organization of a dedicated team caring for the patient. The Contingency Team is a designated group that would be contacted immediately when medical issues develop, so that a plan of action can be developed with all members of the care team involved in the plan, with roles clearly demarcated and specific jobs assigned. Additional staff may be required to assist for a brief period but would be released once emergency has resolved.

Based on the Contingency Team model, all staff members in the Labor and Delivery Unit receive team training through simulations and training modules that are repeated at regular intervals. Drills of obstetric emergencies can be conducted *on site* in labor and delivery unit to help cement key concepts and familiarize staff with their roles. After a critical event, the team debriefs to review what worked well and what did not (Chapter 33, "Principles of Debriefing").

The effectiveness of the Contingency Team model is based on the fundamental concepts of team-based approach: Communication, Situation Monitoring, Mutual Support, and Leadership to improve the patient safety.[4,5]

GOALS

- Improve communication and improve patient outcomes.
- Allow identification and prevention of errors.
- Shorten decision to delivery interval (DDI).

CLINICAL PRACTICE

- Nurses are assigned at the start of each shift for the Contingency Team roles. (See Table 27-1.)
- Specific staff are designated to respond to an emergency; nonassigned staff do not respond to prevent overcrowding and maintain appropriate care levels for other patients.
- Contingency Team role cards with a list of designated duties are used to ensure that all members of a Contingency Team understand their responsibilities on the team.
- Contingency Team is activated when the primary obstetrician makes the decision to call a STAT cesarean delivery (see Fig. 27-1). At that point, the primary nurse activates the **OB Stat Button** (Fig. 27-2) in the labor room, which notifies anesthesiologists, the resource nurse, Contingency Team nurses, obstetric resident, surgical technician, and unit coordinator instantly via an automatic paging system.

The unit coordinator then sends an "OB Emergency" page via the hospital paging system to the anesthesiologist backups to alert them the emergency. The Neonatal Intensive Care Unit (NICU) team is called separately. If the patient has an epidural already in place, a STAT cesarean emergency kit is immediately available to induce surgical block. If the patient does not have an epidural in place, the operating room is prepared for a general anesthesia, or quick spinal if it is possible.

Once the patient is moved to the operating room, Contingency Team members perform their assigned roles. An abbreviated Time Out is then done prior to incision. The Contingency Team workflow is shown in Fig. 27-1.

TABLE 27-1 • The Members of Contingency Team	
Primary obstetrician	Obstetric resident
Anesthesiology attending	Anesthesiology resident
Primary labor room nurse	Backup resource nurse
Operating room nurses 1 and 2	Surgical technician
Resource nurse (charge nurse)	Unit coordinator

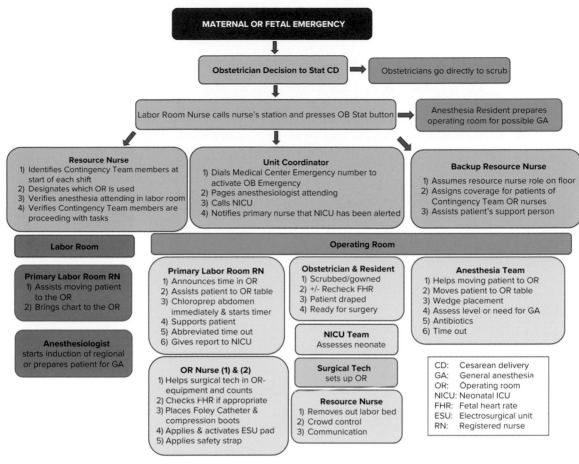

FIGURE 27-1 • Contingency Team workflow.

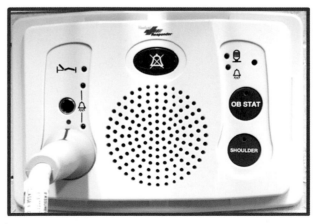

FIGURE 27-2 • OB Stat alarm.

References

1. Kohn L, Corrigan J, Donaldson M. *To Err Is Human: Building a Safer Health System*. Washington, DC: National Academy Press; 1999.

2. Joint Commission. Sentinel event reporting issue 30: Preventing infant death and injury during delivery. https://www.jointcommission.org/-/media/tjc/documents/resources/patient-safety-topics/sentinel-event/sea_30.

3. Pratt S, Mann S, Salisbury M, et al. Impact of CRM-based team training on obstetric outcomes and clinicians' patient safety attitudes. *Jt Comm J Qual Patient Saf*. 2007;33(12):720-725.

4. Guise J, Segel S. Teamwork in obstetric critical care. *Best Pract Res Clin Obstetrics Gynaecol*. 2008;22(5):937-951.

5. Riley W, Begun JW, Meredith L, et al. Integrated approach to reduce perinatal adverse events: standardized processes, interdisciplinary teamwork training, and performance feedback. *Health Serv Res*. 2016;51(6) Part II:2431-2452.

28

Pre-procedure Checklist

Philip E. Hess, MD

The use of a pre-procedure checklist (briefing script) at a huddle, or briefing, provides the opportunity for the team to align to address any missing information and ensure preparation before starting an operation and has been associated with decreases in patient harm. A standardized briefing script can be used prior to entering the operating room to improve communication and enhance patient safety. Our script was revised multiple times based on clinical complications and near-misses. By using this script, we are able to identify *latent errors* prior to entering the operating room.

The briefing script supplements the intraoperative procedural verification (universal protocol, Time out) that occurs immediately before incision. The World Health Organization (WHO) and the Joint Commission (TJC) highly recommend the use of a procedural checklist for verification immediately before incision as a mandatory process.[1] The data from hospitals around the globe have successfully demonstrated that the use of a simple surgical checklist before major operations can help to reduce surgical complications and death.[2]

THE PROCESS OF PRE-PROCEDURE VERIFICATION

Before any invasive procedure, such as cesarean delivery, the surgical team members will gather together for the "**Huddle**." The team members include:

- Obstetric attending
- Obstetric fellow/resident/physician assistant
- Anesthesia attending
- Anesthesia fellow/resident
- Labor and delivery nurse
- Operating room circulator nurse
- Surgical technician

The team members will start by introducing themselves by their first name and roles to help facilitate communication.

BRIEFING SCRIPT

The obstetric pre-procedure checklist is designed specifically for obstetrical patients and was based on identified latent errors that were discovered in our clinical practice. It can be customized to meet any institution's needs.

The Joint Commission had identified our "Briefing Script" for invasive procedures on Labor and Delivery Unit at Beth Israel Deaconess Medical Center[3] (Fig. 28-1) as a best practice during their site visit.

Briefing Script for Invasive Procedures on Labor and Delivery

Briefing occurs at desk immediately before moving to the Operating Room

Present: Primary RN, Attending and Resident anesthesiologist, OB Attending, Scrub tech, OB resident should be identified if not present. Identify all students.

Nurse to ASK	Responsible person to respond
What is everyone's name?	RN faces group: Introduces self, all participate and introduce themselves.
What is patient's name?	RN reads: Label on chart with patient name.
Pertinent Medical History?	RN states: Pertinent medical history, team confirms.
COVID testing complete & Status?	Team states status or looks up results.
What is the procedure being done?	Surgeon states: ALL planned procedures, including contraception.
Indication for the procedure?	Surgeon states: Indication(s).
Planned anesthetic?	Anesthesiologist states: Planned anesthetic (spinal, epidural, CSE, GA, MAC).
Allergies?	RN states: Allergies or NKA, team confirms.
What is planned antibiotic?	Anesthesiologist states: Antibiotic choices, surgeon confirms.
Is Azithromycin indicated?	Surgeon states: Yes (ROM, cervix: ≥4cm) or No
Will a vaginal prep be done?	Surgeon states: Yes or No
Intrapartum Cesarean	RN: -Calculated I&O's -Will magnesium infusion be continued in OR? -Will a push-up be needed? By whom?
What is the IV access?	Anesthesiologist and RN specify: What IV access present, and if sufficient
Is blood available by electronic/Xmatch?	Anesthesiologist answers: YES or NO. Anesthesiologist determines necessity.
Contraindications to uterotonics or TXA?	Anesthesiologist and Surgeon answer: YES or NO.
Is the NICU team needed?	Team answers: NICU will or will NOT be present at delivery
Plan for postoperative pain?	Anesthesiologist states: Neuraxial narcotic, PCA, other
Additional equipment or hovermat?	Team states: What is needed and scrub person confirms. **Hovermat >250 Lbs.**
Is patient in any study?	Investigator describes: What is needed and expected.
Is equipment sterile?	RN and scrub confirm: Sterility of equipment.
Request for clear drapes or birth plan?	RN confirms: Request for clear drape, other.
Are all consents present?	RN states: YES or NO and shows to team all consents present
Is an H&P present?	RN states: YES or NO and shows to team an H&P and 24-hour update
We encourage open communication	All confirm.
Beth Israel Deaconess Medical Center	A briefing must occur before any non-emergent maternal or fetal procedure that is invasive or has potential to become invasive.

FIGURE 28-1 • Briefing script for invasive procedures on labor and delivery. (Reproduced with permission from Briefing script for invasive procedures on labor and delivery (CP-IP 2). Beth Israel Deaconess Medical Center © 2020. Accessed April 2022.) CSE, combined spinal epidural; GA, general anesthesia; H&P, history and physical; I&Os, ins and outs of fluid; IV, intravenous; MAC, monitored anesthesia care; NICU, Neonatal Intensive Care Unit; OR, operating room; PCA, patient-controlled analgesia; RN, registered nurse; ROM, rupture of membranes; TXA, tranexamic acid; Xmatch, blood crossmatch. Source: Beth Israel Deaconess Medical Center. Briefing script for invasive procedures on labor and delivery (CP-IP 2). Used with permission.

References

1. The Joint Commission. The universal protocol for preventing wrong site, wrong procedure, and wrong person surgery™. https://www.jointcommission.org/-/media/tjc/documents/standards/universal-protocol/up_poster1pdf.pdf. Accessed April 2, 2022.

2. World Health Organization. Checklist helps reduce surgical complications, deaths. News release December 11, 2010. www.who.int/news/item/11-12-2010-checklist-helps-reduce-surgical-complications-deaths. Accessed April 2, 2022.

3. Beth Israel Deaconess Medical Center©. Briefing script for invasive procedures on labor and delivery (CP-IP 2), 2020.

29

Whiteboard and Team Meeting

Patsy J. McGuire, MD

BACKGROUND

The labor and delivery unit is a dynamic environment with frequent interruptions and handoffs and a constant pressure to multitask. Along with the emergency department, it is arguably one of the most information-intensive environments where timely multidisciplinary communication is essential to safe and effective operations.[1] Ineffective communication among clinicians has been implicated as a major contributor to adverse obstetric events. Review of closed claims malpractice cases identified communication as a contributing factor in 31% of adverse events where barriers included failure to function as a cohesive team.[2]

Use of a centralized whiteboard for communication, whether dry-erase or electronic, has the potential to aid collaboration and capture a whole picture to decrease adverse events, and optimize clinical and operational management.[3] In Labor and Delivery Unit at Beth Israel Deaconess Medical Center (BIDMC), it has served as an invaluable instrument for communication and management of resources.

AIMS OF THE WHITEBOARD

- To provide a quick high-level overview of the unit's operation
- To share up-to-date individual patient information or relay changes to patient management to all care teams (anesthesia, nursing, obstetrics)
- To improve collaboration and coordination of patient care among all care teams

CLINICAL PRACTICE

The dry-erase whiteboard used for communication measures 6 × 5 feet and is partitioned into columns (Table 29-1). The columns are frequently updated to provide real-time patient information. For example, once a patient delivers, the membranes (M), cervical exam (CX), and time (T) fields are erased and the delivery time and method is noted. Or, if a patient is now going for a cesarean delivery (CD), these fields are erased and "for CD" is written.

SHORTCOMINGS OF THE WHITEBOARD

- Single location to view or update information
- Information is permanently lost once erased from the whiteboard
- Lack of integration with the electronic patient record

TABLE 29-1 • Whiteboard on Labor and Delivery										
Room	Name	GA	MD	RN	GP	M	Cervix	Time	Anesth	MISC
1	S. Smith	32⁶	Abram	Davis	8/1	I	C/L/P	15:30	seen	IUGR, H1
2	B. Held	40³	Bailly	Allen	2/0	AROM	9/100/0	14:25	CSE	IOL, H1
3	K. Day	39²	Fisher	Cassy	3/0	For CD			CSE	H2
4	E. Ellis	38⁶	Cotter	Elsner	3/2	**Delivered at 12:30**			CSE	Labor/ pitocin H1

Column headings (from left to right):
Room number
Patient name
Gestational age
Obstetrician
Nurse
Gravidity and parity
Membrane status: I—Intact
                        SROM—Spontaneous rupture of membrane
                        AROM—Amniotomy, artificial rupture of membrane
Cervical exam: Cervical dilation/enface/station, such as closed/long/posterior
Time of cervical exam: If more than one time point, i.e., there is no changes in cervical exam during the time range
Type of anesthesia: CSE—Combined spinal and epidural; E_{DP}—Epidural with dural puncture; E—Epidural
Miscellaneous: Significant past medical history
                        Significant current obstetric problems
                        Chorioamnionitis
                        Use of antibiotics
                        Intrauterine growth restriction (IUGR)
                        Thrombocytopenia and platelet count
                        Preeclampsia with severe features
                        Induction of labor (IOL) given misoprostol (doses) and whether on oxytocin augmentation
                        Hemorrhage risk evaluation and updates on hemorrhage risk status (H1, H2, H3) (Chapter 34,
                        "Evaluation of Hemorrhage Risks")
                        Other pertinent information

RECENT ADVANCES

Electronic whiteboards are now available in certain institutions, and some have the capability of integrating with the electronic patient record. It can be updated in real time by the different care teams. Obviously, it can be viewed from remote locations by credentialed providers and the data can be stored in a database.

WHITEBOARD AND TEAM MEETING

The team meeting is a moderated and organized meeting for communication. It occurs twice a day in BIDMC's Labor and Delivery Unit at 10:30 and 22:30. When the acuity is high, the leadership can decide to add another one at any time (Fig. 29-1).

- Goal of the team meeting
  - Establishing a culture of communication at BIDMC[4]
  - Empowering all healthcare providers to be able to speak up if they have any concerns about patient safety
  - Improving the quality and safety of obstetrical care
- Where will the team meeting be held?
  - At the Whiteboard by the nursing station
- Who will attend?
  - Obstetricians

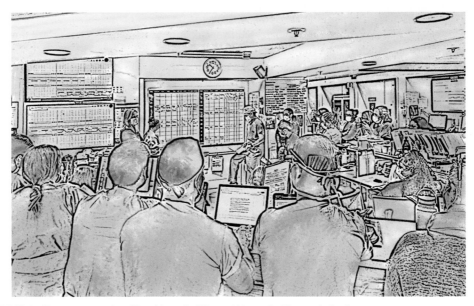

FIGURE 29-1 • The team meeting. (Graphic art by Mingwei Li, used with permission.)

- ○ Obstetric Anesthesiologists
- ○ Obstetric Nurses
- ○ Resource Nurse on Labor and Delivery
- ○ Resource Nurses on Postpartum floors
- ○ Hospital bed facilitator
- ○ The unit coordinator
- ○ One representative from Neonatal ICU
- • Who will lead the team meeting?
  - ○ The resource nurse on Labor and Delivery
- • How are patients presented at the team meeting?
  - ○ The patient's primary nurse presents the case using the "Team Meeting Script" (Box 29-1)

BOX 29-1 • Team Meeting Script

Patient name
Parity
Gestational age
Diagnosis
Pertinent medical history
Pertinent medications
Last vaginal exam
Obstetric hemorrhage risk (H1, H2, H3)
Fetal heart rate category
Plan of care
For postpartum patients: pertinent neonatal history, and hypoglycemia screening

- Discussion of plan of care and any concerns
  - All team members are expected to speak and raise any concerns or ask questions, including anesthesia concerns and hemorrhage risks
- At the end of the team meeting, the Resource nurse reads **"the Safety Pearl of the Week"** with brief discussion (Chapter 30, "Safety Pearls")

References

1. Aronsky D, Jones I, Lanaghan K, et al. Supporting patient care in the emergency department with a computerized whiteboard system. *J Am Med Inform Assoc.* 2008;15:184-194.

2. Austin N, Goldhaber-Fiebert S, Daniels K, et al. Building comprehensive strategies for obstetric safety: simulation drills and communication. *Anesth Analg.* 2016;123(5):1181-1190.

3. Xiao Y, Schenkel S, Faraj S, et al. What whiteboard in a trauma center operating suite can teach us about emergency department communication. *Ann Emerg Med.* 2007;50(4):387-395.

4. Pratt S, Mann S, Salisbury M, et al. Impact of CRM-based team training on obstetric outcomes and clinicians' patient safety attitudes. *Jt Comm J Qual Patient Saf.* 2007;33(12):720-725.

30

Safety Pearls

Colin B. Jackson, MD

BACKGROUND

Labor and Delivery (L&D) is a high-acuity, fast-paced work environment, frequently with a large, shifting workforce. In this setting, it can be difficult for personnel to stay current on best practices and updated policies. As policies are introduced or changed, there is variable exposure to the changes and uptake of the novel, desired behaviors. Communication with this type of workforce in this environment can be difficult. While email seems an obvious choice to communicate with the large workforce, we know that high email volume and email fatigue prevents it from being an effective way to disseminate essential updates.[1] In-person communication is limited in scope as only a small proportion of personnel are present during any shift.

The Safety Pearl is a 60-second or shorter announcement that occurs at the end of each Team Meeting (Chapter 29, "Whiteboard and Team Meeting"). The format was developed to address the above difficulties in communication. It provides timely, accurate, and succinct information to the clinical workforce on L&D.[2] It provides a standardized, consistent message that is easy to repeat across multiple shifts. It also reaches a sizeable portion of the clinical workforce as it is repeated twice a day for an entire week at Team Meeting. This format leads to most personnel having at least one exposure to the critical update (Fig. 30-1).

GOALS

- Communicate to all staff on L&D key learning points from patient safety events.
- Reinforce a culture of safety by spotlighting patient safety twice a day during Team Meetings.
- Encourage standardization of care by highlighting correct practice as a way to improve patient safety.[3]

CLINICAL PRACTICE

- Safety Pearl topics are identified through many channels:
  - Recommendations during a monthly interdisciplinary meeting reviewing policies.
  - Patient safety reports from monthly Department of Obstetrics and Gynecology Quality Assurance/Quality Improvement meeting.
  - Outreach from fellows and residents working on L&D.
  - Input from L&D nurses.
  - Repeating Safety Pearls on core safety concepts.

Safety Pearl
Week of 12/20/2022

Topic: Communicating towards consensus

When a disagreement occurs about the safest plan of care for the patient, effective communication follows the DESC script. "D" - Describe the specific situation with objective descriptions. "E" - Express your concern for patient safety. "S" - Suggest other alternatives and seek agreement. "C" - Consensus is the goal of the conversation. Utilize the chain of command as needed.

Background
Team training based communication tools like SBAR (Situation-Background-Assessment-Recommendation) or DESC may be helpful in guiding difficult conversations. In some situations this may be difficult or inappropriate. In these situations, the Obstetric Clinical Conflict Resolution guideline may serve as a resource to move the team toward mutual understanding.

CP-OB 28 Obstetric Clinical Conflict Resolution describes the process for all obstetric healthcare personnel (nurse, physician, midlevel, perinatal scrub technician, unit coordinator, patient care technician) to resolve conflict when there is a question or concern regarding patient care, patient safety, or uncertainty of how to proceed in a clinical situation.

Reference
CP-OB 28 Obstetric Clinical Conflict Resolution

FIGURE 30-1 • Sample Safety Pearl format.

- The topic is distilled down to no more than two key takeaways, which can be read in less than 60 seconds.
- Each Safety Pearl is reviewed by a nurse and physician to ensure accuracy, with a final review by the L&D medical director.
- The Safety Pearl is read at the end of the Team Meeting, a twice a day meeting that brings together the nursing, anesthesia, and obstetric teams to discuss every patient on the floor.
- Safety Pearls are based on written policies. Each Safety Pearl is accompanied by a resource sheet with additional information and reference to the policy and potentially relevant literature.
- Topics are diverse; some examples are as follows:
  - Review Maternal Early Warning System criteria and desired clinical response.
  - Announce changes to visitor policy with changes in COVID-19 incidence.
  - Describe changes to criteria for evaluation of hemorrhage risks (H-Score).
  - Identify the location of resuscitative cesarean delivery kit to be used during maternal cardiac arrest and reminder of how to activate code team.
  - List recent medication duplications and changes to the ordering system to address this risk.
  - State conflict resolution scripts and how to utilize the chain of command.

References

1. Paul IM, Levi BH. Metastasis of email at an academic medical center. *JAMA Pediatr*. 2014;168(3):290.

2. Levine D, Gadivemula J, Kutaimy R, Kamatam S, Sarvadevabatla N, Lohia P. Analysis of patient safety messages delivered and received during clinical rounds. *BMJ Open Qual*. 2020;9(3):e000869.

3. Clinical guidelines and standardization of practice to improve outcomes: ACOG Committee Opinion, Number 792. *Obstet Gynecol*. 2019;134(4):e122-e125.

31

Quality Indicators

Anna Moldysz, MD

Yunping Li, MD

Philip E. Hess, MD

BACKGROUND

"No monitoring, no improvement." Measuring quality indicators is necessary for improving patient safety and quality of care. To assess quality of care, effective and meaningful indicators must be defined, monitored, and reported. Unfortunately, consensus indicators are lacking at a national level.

Some of the organizations that define quality in healthcare are:

- **CMS**—Centers for Medicare & Medicaid Services
- **TJC**—The Joint Commission
- **CDC**—Centers for Disease Control and Prevention

Initiatives to improve quality in anesthesia will continue to significantly impact and shape practice. The Anesthesia Quality Institute (AQI) was established in 2008. The AQI created the National Anesthesia Clinical Outcomes Registry (NACOR) in 2010. The vision of the AQI is as follows:

- Improve quality care of patients.
- Lower anesthesia mortality.
- Lower anesthesia adverse incidents.

Similar initiatives at the subspecialty level led the Society for Obstetric Anesthesia and Perinatology (SOAP) to create the Serious Complication Repository (SCORE) in 2004. This data collection captured the incidence of serious obstetric anesthesia–related complications,[1] including:

- Maternal death
- Cardiac arrest
- Myocardial infarction
- Epidural abscess/meningitis
- Epidural hematoma
- Serious neurologic injury
- Aspiration
- Failed intubation
- High neuraxial block
- Anaphylaxis
- Respiratory arrest in labor suite
- Unrecognized spinal catheter

NUMBERS AND VOLUME

Obstetric anesthesia service should, at a minimum, be able to report the monthly and yearly number of procedures.

Labor Analgesia

- Combined spinal and epidural (CSE)
- Epidural
- Dural puncture epidural (DPE)
- Intrathecal catheters
- Epidural replacement (second neuraxial procedure)
- Patient-controlled analgesia (PCA)

Cesarean Delivery and Other Operative Procedures

- Labor converted to cesarean delivery (CD)
- Failed labor epidural conversion to anesthesia for cesarean (requiring either endotracheal tube or laryngeal mask airway [LMA] after neuraxial)
- Scheduled cesarean delivery (cesarean no labor analgesia)
- External cephalic version (ECV)
- Dilation and curettage (D&C)
- Tubal ligation
- Postpartum hemorrhage
- Cardioversion

Type of anesthesia for Cesarean Delivery

- CSE
- Epidural
- Spinal
- DPE
- Intrathecal catheters
- General anesthesia (GA)
- Monitored anesthesia care (MAC)

Other Parameters

- Number of patients with vaginal delivery
- Number of patients with neuraxial analgesia for vaginal delivery
- Peripheral nerve blocks
- Arterial line
- Central line
- Blood transfusion and products
- ICU admission

OBSTETRIC ANESTHESIA QUALITY INDICATORS (TABLE 31-1)

TABLE 31-1 • Obstetric Anesthesia Quality Indicators

Indicators	Definition	Incidence	References
General anesthesia rate[2,3]	$\dfrac{CD\ requiring\ GA}{Total\ CD} \times 100$	Overall CD ≤5% Emergent or urgent CD <10%	SOAP Centers of Excellence[2,4]
The rate of failed intubation for GA for CD	$\dfrac{Number\ of\ failed\ intubation}{Total\ number\ of\ GA\ for\ CD}$	1/379 Or 1/533	Obstetric anesthetic practice in the UK[5] SCORE Project[1]
Aspiration	$\dfrac{Number\ of\ patient\ aspirated}{Total\ number\ of\ anesthetics}$	0/256,795	SCORE Project[1]
Unintentional dural puncture (UDP) rate	$\dfrac{Number\ of\ UDP}{Total\ neuraxial\ for\ labor\ and\ CD} \times 100$	≤2%	SOAP Centers of Excellence[2]
The rate of high neuraxial block causing loss of consciousness	$\dfrac{Number\ of\ high\ neuraxial\ block}{Total\ neuraxial\ for\ labor\ and\ CD}$	1/6667 Or 1/4366	Obstetric anesthetic practice in the UK[5] SCORE Project[1]
The rate of failed labor epidural requiring replacement	$\dfrac{Number\ of\ replacement}{Total\ neuraxial\ for\ labor} \times 100$	5-7%	Reference[6]
Failed neuraxial anesthesia that required an alternate technique for CD	$\dfrac{Number\ of\ failed\ neuraxial}{Total\ neuraxial\ for\ CD} \times 100$	1.7%	SCORE Project[1]
Unrecognized intrathecal (IT) catheter	$\dfrac{Number\ of\ unrecognized\ IT\ catheter}{Total\ epidural\ \&\ CSE\ for\ CD\ \&\ labor}$	1/15,435	SCORE Project[1]
Anesthesia-related serious neurologic injury	$\dfrac{Anesthesia-related\ neurologic\ injury}{Total\ neuraxial\ for\ labor\ and\ CD}$	1/35,923	SCORE Project[1]
Medication errors	$\dfrac{Number\ of\ medication\ errors}{Total\ patient\ received\ anesthesia}$	Not available	Not available
Administration of antibiotics for CD	Documentation of antibiotics administration	100%	
Postpartum visit	All patients who received anesthesia seen within 48 hours of delivery	100%	
Quality of recovery scores after elective CD	ObsQoR-11: nausea and vomiting, shivering, dizzy, feeling in control, been comfortable, moderate pain, severe pain, able to hold baby, able to feed baby, mobilizing independently, can look after personal hygiene. Assess at 24 hours after delivery	0-10 scale	ObsQoR-11[7]

SERIOUS COMPLICATIONS

Severe maternal morbidity (SMM) is a major adverse outcome leading to maternal harm.[8] CDC updated the list of 21 SMM indicators and corresponding ICD codes.[9] These 21 SMM may not directly relate to obstetric anesthesia practice; however, anesthetic care can be a contributing factor to some of these outcomes.

- Cardiac arrest/ventricular fibrillation
- Aneurysm
- Conversion of cardiac rhythm
- Disseminated intravascular coagulation (DIC)
- Acute myocardial infarction
- Acute renal failure
- Eclampsia
- Heart failure/arrest during surgery or procedure
- Acute respiratory distress syndrome and respiratory arrest necessitating naloxone reversal or intubation
- Puerperal cerebrovascular disorders
- Pulmonary edema/acute heart failure
- Severe anesthesia complications including (with ICD-10 code):
  - Maternal death
  - Aspiration pneumonitis due to anesthesia during labor and delivery (O89.01 and O74.0)
  - Other pulmonary complications of anesthesia during labor and delivery (O74.1)
  - Cardiac complications of anesthesia during labor and delivery (O74.2 and O89.1)
  - Central nervous system complications of anesthesia during the puerperium (O89.2)
  - Epidural abscess/meningitis (O89.5—other complications of spinal and epidural anesthesia during the puerperium)
  - Epidural hematoma (O89.5—other complications of spinal and epidural anesthesia during the puerperium)
  - Failed intubation (O89.6—failed or difficult intubation for anesthesia during the puerperium)
  - High neuraxial block necessitating intubation (O89.09)
  - Local anesthetic systemic toxicity (LAST) (O89.3—toxic reaction to local anesthesia during the puerperium)
- Acute amniotic fluid embolism
- Sepsis
- Shock
- Sickle cell disease with crisis
- Air and thrombotic embolism
- Blood product transfusion
- Hysterectomy
- Temporary tracheostomy
- Ventilation

References

1. D'Angelo R, Smiley RM, Riley ET, et al. Serious complications related to obstetric anesthesia. The serious complication repository project of the Society of Obstetric Anesthesia and Perinatology. *Anesthesiology*. 2014;120(6):1505-1512.
2. The Society for Obstetric Anesthesia and Perinatology, Centers of Excellence. https://www.soap.org/centers-of-excellence_program. Accessed April 2022.
3. Carvalho B, Mhyre J. Centers of excellence for anesthesia care of obstetric patients. *Anesth Analg*. 2019;128(5):844-846.
4. Palanisamy A, Mitani AA, Tsen LC. General anesthesia for cesarean delivery at a tertiary hospital from 2000 to 2005: a retrospective analysis and 10-year update. *Int J Obstet Anesth*. 2011;20:10-16.
5. Bamber JH, Lucas DN, Plaat F, et al. Obstetric anaesthetic practice in the UK: a descriptive analysis of the national obstetric anaesthetic database 2009-14. *Br J Anaesth*. 2020;125(4):580-587.
6. Pan PH, Bogard TD, Owen MD. Incidence and characteristics of failures in obstetric neuraxial analgesia and anesthesia: a retrospective analysis of 19,259 deliveries. *Int J Obstet Anesth*. 2004;13(4):227-233.
7. Ciechanowicz S, Setty T, Robson E, et al. Development and evaluation of an obstetric quality-of-recovery score (ObsQoR-11) after elective caesarean delivery. *Br J Anaesth*. 2019;122(1):69-78.
8. The American College of Obstetricians and Gynecologists. Severe maternal morbidity: screening and review. September 2016. https://www.acog.org/clinical/clinical-guidance/obstetric-care-consensus/articles/2016/09/severe-maternal-morbidity-screening-and-review. Accessed April 2022.
9. Centers for Disease Control and Prevention. How does CDC identify severe maternal morbidity? https://www.cdc.gov/reproductivehealth/maternalinfanthealth/smm/severe-morbidity-ICD.htm. Accessed April 2022.

32

Transition of Care

Yunping Li, MD

BACKGROUND

The Labor and Delivery Unit is characterized by collaboration between multiple teams, high information output, and rapidly evolving changes in patient conditions. A comprehensive handoff, i.e., transition of care, facilitates communication among teams, continuity of care, and patient safety. Accreditation Council for Graduate Medical Education (ACGME) emphasizes the proper training of "Structured and Effective Transition of Care."[1,2]

PROCESS OF HANDOFF

When Does the Handoff Occur?

- Shift changes
- When provider(s) changes during a surgery
- When the patient is transferred to the Postanesthesia Care Unit (PACU) or Intensive Care Unit (ICU); Chapter 53, "Postanesthetic Care"

Who Needs a Handoff?

- Every patient in Labor and Delivery Unit
- Every patient in PACU
- Any patients who need follow-up on the postpartum floors or as an outpatient
- Any antepartum patients who may need potential urgent anesthesia care
- Any patient admitted to ICU

How to Handoff?

The comprehensive handoff includes "General Information" and "Specific Information" (Table 32-1).

TABLE 32-1 • Handoff Script for Obstetric Patients	
General Information	**Specific Information**
• Age • Gravidity and parity • Gestational age • Allergies • Body Mass Index (BMI) • Airway exam • Labor epidural including information regarding difficult placement, breakthrough pain management, etc. • Labor course, category of fetal heart rate tracing	• If preeclamptic, details of severe features and related laboratory results • If trial of labor after cesarean (TOLAC), indication for prior cesarean • If high risk of hemorrhage (H2 and H3), reasons for H2 and H3 • If thrombocytopenic, the trend of platelet counts • If cesarean delivery (CD), intraoperative information and plan for post CD analgesia • Other significant medical history

H1, average risk of obstetric hemorrhage; H2, above average risk of bleeding; H3, significant risk of bleeding (Chapter 34, "Evaluation of Hemorrhage Risks").

References

1. VI.E.3. Transitions of care. ACGME program requirements for graduate medical education in anesthesiology 2022. https://www.acgme.org/globalassets/pfassets/programrequirements/040_anesthesiology_2022.pdf. Accessed in December 2022.
2. Agarwala AV, Lane-Fall MB, Greilich PE, et al. Consensus recommendations for the conduct, training, implementation, and research of perioperative handoffs. *Anesth Anal.* 2019;128(5):e71-e78.

33

Principles of Debriefing

Liana Zucco, MD, MBBS

Debriefing is the practice of facilitated discussion between participants—reflecting on actions and thought processes. Distinct from feedback, or the one-way transfer of information, debriefing is a powerful tool that enables reflection, enhances operational efficiency, and improves clinical performance and interprofessional dynamics.[1,2] Debriefing has increasingly been incorporated into healthcare settings, in training, and within real-time clinical practice. In obstetrics specifically, the implementation of routine debriefing programs has demonstrated improvement in clinical outcomes and is therefore recommended by the American College of Obstetrics and Gynecology as a tool to help prepare for and manage clinical emergencies.[3]

PURPOSE OF DEBRIEFING

- To reflect on important components of routine care or a critical event, create a shared mental model, understand the thought processes leading to actions
- To evaluate clinical workflow efficiency, facilitate interprofessional training, review clinical performance metrics, and promote continuous improvement, e.g., identify hazards within the workplace and propose risk mitigation strategies
- To foster a culture of safety and cultivate an environment which acknowledges psychological burden and promotes provider wellbeing[4]

HOW TO DEBRIEF

Healthcare teams should consider the following when establishing a debriefing program in their organization:

- A list of events that would trigger a debrief
- The purpose of the debrief
- The participants, facilitator(s), timing, and format
- The content to be covered, the structure of the debriefing session, and the follow-up processes

These are summarized in Table 33-1. Furthermore, great care must be taken to appreciate the potential sensitive nature of debriefing, given preexisting concerns of punitive behavior and psychological distress.[4]

Debriefing in Practice

Table 33-2 is an example of the framework and script currently in use in our institution, following adverse events that occur during simulation training and real clinical adverse events.

TABLE 33-1 • What to Consider When Debriefing in Obstetrics		
Trigger	Specific critical events (e.g., maternal death, hemorrhage, unplanned general anesthesia)	
Purpose	Should be predetermined and agreed among the group Often impacts how the remainder of the debrief is organized	
Timing	**Following an adverse clinical encounter:** • Immediately; "hot" • Within a few hours or days; "warm" • Several days afterward; "cold"	**After routine clinical care:** • Per patient or end of the day **After an educational session:** • Postsimulation training
Participants	**Clinical staff:** • All physicians and nursing staff (e.g., obstetrics, anesthesia, neonatology) • Therapists, pharmacists, technologists • Any other relevant clinical support staff, e.g., operating room staff	
	Nonclinical staff: • Hospital or departmental Quality and Safety or governance member • Other: social worker, mental health team member, clergy, unit coordinators	
	All staff members involved should be invited, all levels. • Organizations should respect the decision of those who do not wish to participate	
Location	**In-person:** • A protected space, free from distraction • The exact site of the adverse event • An informal space: e.g., the hallway or on the labor and delivery unit	**Virtual platform:** • Enables larger participant group presence • Strict patient/provider data protection measures required
Content/ Structure	**Key elements that should be present within each debrief include:** • Vocalization of the intended purpose of the debrief • Establishment of rules or code of conduct • Establishment of a shared mental model • Use of reflective techniques (e.g., open-ended questions or silence) • Ensuring awareness of support resources **The use of a framework provides a focus to the discussion:** • +/delta model, three-phase approaches (e.g., Reaction-Analysis-Summary) • Multiphase approaches (e.g., PEARLS, TeamGAINS) • Unpublished technique, but structured and site-specific	
Tools	To facilitate the session, maintain structure, support documentation, and encourage supportive language around debriefing; e.g., **a cognitive aid (checklist) or a script**	

Debriefing frameworks[5]: PEARLS, Promoting Excellence and Reflective Learning in Simulation; TeamGAINS, Team-Guided team self-correction, Advocacy-Inquiry, and Systemic-constructivist.

TABLE 33-2 • Debriefing Script—An Example from the BIDMC

The following are read aloud by the debriefing facilitator:

Statement of Intent	**The purpose of this debrief is to:** • Provide a supportive space for each person involved in the case to discuss • Review the events and establish a shared mental model of what happened • DO NOT critically review the details of the event • Improve performance as a team and the care we provide • Foster a culture of safety within the organization
Basic Rules	**This is a blameless environment** • We encourage everyone to speak up and participate actively • Everyone's voice is valuable • Try not to interrupt others, be respectful of all team members • Do not record this meeting, leave electronic devices off, if possible • This is a confidential discussion and not part of the medical record
Expression of Gratitude	Thank you to everyone who helped in the care of this patient
Agenda	We will use the following structure to guide this debrief [enter chosen framework] This session will last approx. [enter duration] We will begin by: • Reviewing the case, incl. the clinical course and management steps • The discussion might include crisis resources management principles, e.g., defined leadership, situational awareness, anticipation of the next step, clear closed-loop communication, distribution of workload, and allocation of attention to tasks of importance We will aim to discuss: • What went well? • What did not go well? • General impressions and reflections of case (incl. provider reactions) • If any safety concerns, risks, or hazards were identified • What are the opportunities for systemic change?

BIDMC, Beth Israel Deaconess Medical Center.

References

1. Gardner R. Introduction to debriefing. *Semin Perinatol [Internet]*. 2013;37(3):166-174. http://dx.doi.org/10.1053/j.semperi.2013.02.008.
2. Brindle ME, Henrich N, Foster A, et al. Implementation of surgical debriefing programs in large health systems: an exploratory qualitative analysis. *BMC Health Serv Res*. 2018;18(1):210.
3. American College of Obstetricians and Gynecologists. Preparing for clinical emergencies in obstetrics and gynecology. Committee Opinion No. 590. *Obstet Gynecol*. 2014;123:722-725.
4. Rudolph JW, Simon R, Dufresne RL, Raemer DB. There's no such thing as "nonjudgmental" debriefing: a theory and method for debriefing with good judgment. *Simul Healthc*. 2006;1(1):49-55.
5. Endacott R, Gale T, O'Connor A, Dix S. Frameworks and quality measures used for debriefing in team-based simulation: a systematic review. *BMJ Simul Technol Enhanc Learn*. 2019;5(2):61-72.

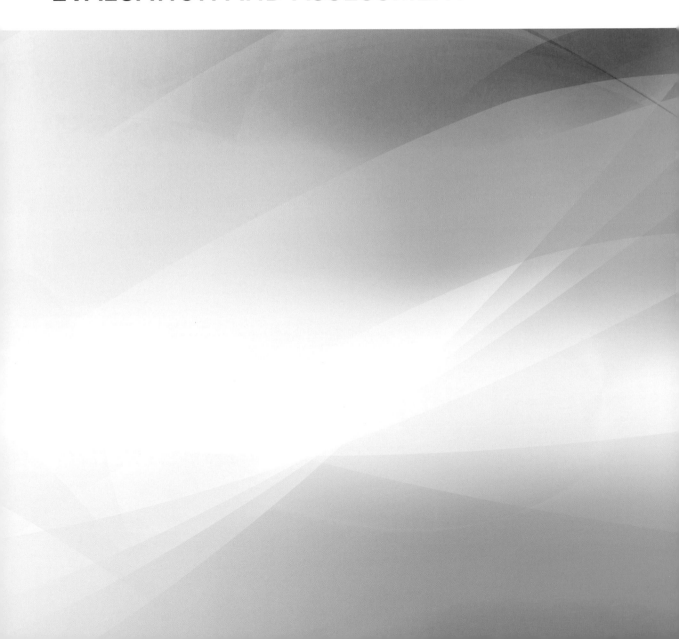

PART V
EVALUATION AND ASSESSMENT

34

Evaluation of Hemorrhage Risks

Philip E. Hess, MD

Obstetric hemorrhage is one of the leading causes of preventable maternal morbidity and mortality worldwide.[1] Numerous hemorrhage risk evaluation tools are available; however, there remains a gap in resources and implementation. In a retrospective cohort analysis of multicenter databases including 56,903 women, composite maternal morbidity occurred at a rate of 2.2%, 8%, and 11.9% within low-risk, medium-risk, and high-risk groups, respectively.[2] The goal of establishing an evaluation tool for obstetric hemorrhage is to identify patient populations who could benefit from risk-reducing interventions.

Three published risk-assessment tools include:

- The Association of Women's Health, Obstetric and Neonatal Nurses (AWHONN) hemorrhage risk-prediction tool[3]
- The American College of Obstetricians and Gynecologists (ACOG) Safe Motherhood Initiative[4]
- California Maternal Quality Care Collaborative (CMQCC) obstetric hemorrhage risk factor assessment screen[1]

Evaluation of obstetric hemorrhage risk is *an ongoing process*. In our medical center, risk evaluation occurs at admission, during labor, postpartum; current risk (H-score) is presented at "Team Meetings" (Chapter 29, "Whiteboard and Team Meeting"). Understanding that the risk factors can escalate during labor is critical for clinical preparation and management.

The unique advantage of risk-assessment tool at Beth Israel Deaconess Medical Center (BIDMC) is linked to actions and preparation (Table 34-1).[5]

TABLE 34-1 • Beth Israel Deaconess Medical Center Obstetric Hemorrhage Risk Evaluation Tool[5]	
Average Risk: H1	
• No risk factors listed in H2 or H3 • No known bleeding disorders	**Actions** • Type and screen
Above Average Risk: H2	
• Previous cesarean delivery • Prior uterine surgery • Multiple gestation • Five or more previous vaginal delivery • History of postpartum hemorrhage • Body Mass Index >40 • Large uterine fibroid (>6 cm) • Macrosomia (Estimated fetal weight >5000 g) • Polyhydramnios (Amniotic Fluid Index >24) • Five or more doses of misoprostol • IV oxytocin for >24 continuous hours • Chorioamnionitis • Operative vaginal delivery • Magnesium • Second stage of labor >3 hours • Consider changing risk group to significant if three or more average risk factors coexist	**Actions** • Type and screen—identify whether a candidate for electronic crossmatch • If not a candidate for electronic crossmatch, the patient is H3[a] • Identify as "H2" at the team meeting and/or pre-procedure briefing • All care providers review the Obstetrical Hemorrhage Protocol
Significant Risk: H3	
• Placenta previa, low-lying placenta • Placental accreta spectrum • Hematocrit <30 and other risk factors • Platelet <100,000/mm³ • Active vaginal bleeding • Known coagulopathy • Suspected placenta abruption • Retained placenta	**Actions** • Type and crossmatch (if electronic not appropriate) • Obtain the second IV access • Identify as "H3" at the team meeting and/or pre-procedure briefing • Ensure uterotonics available at delivery • Ensure hemorrhage cart available and stocked • Review MEWS[b] criteria for activation • All care providers review the Obstetrical Hemorrhage Protocol

[a]*The presence of red cell blood antibodies does not increase risk of postpartum hemorrhage. However, obtaining Type and Cross is recommended given increased difficulty with crossmatch.*
[b]*MEWS, maternal early warning system.*
Source: *Reproduced with permission from PPGD CP-OB 55 Evaluation for obstetrical hemorrhage risk tool 2016. © Beth Israel Deaconess Medical Center. Accessed April 2022.*

References

1. California Maternity Quality Care Collaborative (CMQCC). Obstetric hemorrhage toolkit version 3.0—Appendix K: obstetric hemorrhage risk factor assessment screen. Accessed April 2022.

2. Colalillo EL, Sparks AD, Phillips JM, et al. Obstetric hemorrhage risk assessment tool predicts composite maternal morbidity. *Sci Rep*. 2021;11:14709.

3. Association of Women's Health, Obstetric and Neonatal Nurses (AWHONN). Postpartum hemorrhage (PPH) risk assessment Table 1.1 Accessed April 2022.

4. The American College of Obstetricians and Gynecologists (ACOG). Safe Motherhood Initiative. Obstetric hemorrhage bundle. Risk assessment table: labor & delivery admission and intrapartum. Accessed April 2022.

5. Beth Israel Deaconess Medical Center. PPGD CP-OB 55 evaluation for obstetrical hemorrhage risk tool 2016. Accessed April 2022. Use with permission.

35

Blood Type and Crossmatch

Yunping Li, MD

PRACTICE AT BIDMC

Our institutional practice is to have all parturients have an active blood sample in the Blood Bank. The following indications of blood typing and crossmatching are based on risk factors for postpartum hemorrhage according to integrated recommendations from the American College of Obstetrics and Gynecology,[1] California Maternal Quality Care Collaborative,[2] and the guidelines of Beth Israel Deaconess Medical Center (BIDMC) at Boston. Individualized recommendations for type and screen or crossmatch are based on these relative risks (Chapter 34, "Evaluation of Hemorrhage Risks").

TYPE AND SCREEN

Patients who require an active type and screen include:

- Significant uterine surgery ×3 or greater
- Previous postpartum hemorrhage
- Known significant uterine fibroids (>6 cm)
- Multiple gestations
- Grand multiparous (>4 term deliveries)
- Macrosomia (estimated fetal weight >5000 g)
- Polyhydramnios (Amniotic fluid index >24)
- Known antibodies in the blood
- Placenta previa
- Abruption in current pregnancy
- Concern for abnormal placentation
- Known coagulopathy
- Platelet <100,000/mm^3
- Hematocrit <28%
- Body Mass Index (BMI) >40 kg/m^2
- Induction of labor used five or more doses of misoprostol
- Intravenous oxytocin >24 continuous hours
- Chorioamnionitis
- The second stage of labor >3 hours

TYPE AND CROSSMATCH

Patients who require an active type and crossmatch:

- Placenta previa, abruption, placenta accreta spectrum (accreta, increta, and percreta)
- Active postpartum hemorrhage and hemodynamic instability
- Known antibodies (except Rhogam antibodies)
- Retained placenta
- Known coagulopathy

CONSIDERATIONS FOR RHOGAM

- After Rhogam administration, the patient will not be "Electronic Crossmatch Eligible" due to the presence of the Rhogam (anti-D) antibody. The blood bank needs **75 minutes** to perform blood type and screen. Identification of Rhogam antibody is the most common reason of delaying the cesarean delivery.
- Page/call the Blood Bank if you have any questions.

References

1. The American College of Obstetricians and Gynecologists (ACOG). Safe Motherhood Initiative. Obstetric hemorrhage bundle. Risk assessment table: labor & delivery admission and intrapartum. Accessed April 2022.
2. California Maternity Quality Care Collaborative (CMQCC). Obstetric hemorrhage toolkit version 3.0—Appendix K: obstetric hemorrhage risk factor assessment screen. Accessed April 2022.

36

NPO Guidelines

Maria C. Borrelli, DO

NPO means "nothing by mouth", from the Latin nil per os. Our guidelines for food intake during labor have integrated the recommendations from the American Society of Anesthesiologists practice guidelines for obstetric anesthesia and the Society for Obstetric Anesthesia and Perinatology task force.[1–3]

DURING LABOR WITH LABOR EPIDURAL

- Moderate amounts of **clear liquids** for uncomplicated laboring women. Clear liquids must be nonparticulate, e.g., water, carbonated beverages, sports drinks, fruit juices (no pulps), tea, and black coffee.
- Avoid milk, cream in the tea and coffee.
- Solid food should be avoided.
- Patients with increased risks for operative delivery have further restrictions on food intake.

ELECTIVE CESAREAN DELIVERY

- Last regular meal up to 8 hours prior.
- Light, low-fat snacks (e.g., crackers, one slice of dry toast) up to 6 hours prior.
- Clear liquids (carbonated, nonparticulate 45-g carbohydrate beverage) up to 2 hours prior.
- Patients with increased aspiration risks (morbid obesity, long-standing diabetes, difficult airway) may have further restrictions on food intake.

UNPLANNED CESAREAN DELIVERY

- NPO as soon as the decision for cesarean delivery is made.
- Depending on the urgency of delivery, anesthesia and obstetric team decide timing based on last intake.
- May utilize ultrasound to assess gastric content.

References

1. Practice Guidelines for Obstetric Anesthesia: An Updated Report by the American Society of Anesthesiologists Task Force on Obstetric Anesthesia and the Society for Obstetric Anesthesia and Perinatology. *Anesthesiology.* 2016;124(2):270-300.

2. Considerations for NPO Guidelines and Gastric Emptying during Labor. SOAP Task Force for OB/GYN Continuing Education; 2019.

3. Beth Israel Deaconess Medical Center. PPGD CP-PP 22 enhanced recovery after cesarean delivery (CarePath). Accessed April 2022. Use with permission.

37

Anesthesia Consultation

Philip E. Hess, MD

PURPOSE

Recognition of significant risks for anesthetic or obstetric complications should encourage an anesthesia consult.[1] The consultation allows for advance planning and preparation; helps to determine what additional tests, consults, or treatment should be obtained; and facilitates early and ongoing multidisciplinary communication, if indicated. Antepartum obstetric anesthesia consults should be obtained after fetal viability, but early enough in gestation to allow for scheduling of appropriate diagnostic tests (generally between 24- and 34-weeks' gestation). The availability of bedside point-of-care ultrasound can aid in patient counseling (e.g., neuraxial ultrasound for scoliosis or high body mass index [BMI]).

REASONS TO REQUEST AN ANESTHESIA CONSULT[2]

- Pre-pregnancy BMI >45 or current weight over 300 lbs
- Severe facial and neck edema or malformation
- Extremely short stature
- Abnormally short neck (or after a surgery with fusion of the neck)
- Difficulty opening the mouth
- Large thyroid
- Severe asthma
- Serious medical or obstetrical complications, including, but not limited to, medical conditions such as:
  - Cardiac (e.g., valvular stenosis or moderate to severe regurgitation, significant arrhythmia, cardiomyopathy)
  - Pulmonary, including severe asthma
  - Neurologic
  - Hematologic
  - Spine (history of spinal surgery, significant scoliosis, or unstable lumbar pain syndrome)
  - Any other significant problem that the obstetrician or patient believes could negatively impact the safe or effective administration of anesthesia for delivery
- History of complications with anesthetics
- History of chronic use of prescription pain medicines or buprenorphine (subutex or suboxone) prior or during pregnancy
- Current use of anticoagulant medications

Consultation for inpatients may be considered with:

- Pregnancy-associated hypertensive disorders (preeclampsia with severe features, HELLP [hemolysis, elevated liver enzymes, and low platelets] syndrome)
- Placental abruption
- Placenta previa
- Abnormal placentation (accreta, increta, percreta)
- Platelet count less than 100,000/mm^3
- Plan for nonobstetric surgery during pregnancy
- Serious conditions that may necessitate emergency cesarean delivery

HOW TO OBTAIN AN ANESTHESIA CONSULT

Call extension 123-456-7890 to leave a message (24/7). Or you can email AnesthesiaOBConsults@yourinstitute.edu

The following information is needed:

- Patient name, medical record number, and contact information
- Obstetrician's name and contact information
- Indication for consult
- Estimated delivery date
- Whether interpreter is necessary

An anesthesiologist (a senior resident or fellow, with an attending physician) will see the patient on Labor and Delivery Unit for the consult, or on the antepartum floor if the patient is currently admitted.

- There is no fee for this consult.
- The anesthesiologist will write a note in the online medical record and forward this note to the obstetrician. If needed, further communication with the obstetrician of any additional tests, consults, therapies will be made.

References

1. Practice guidelines for obstetric anesthesia. An updated report by the American Society of Anesthesiologists task force on obstetric anesthesia and the Society for Obstetric Anesthesia and Perinatology. *Anesthesiology*. 2016;124(2):270-300.
2. American College of Obstetricians and Gynecologists. Practice Bulletin No. 209: Obstetric analgesia and anesthesia. *Obstet Gynecol*. 2019;133(3):e208-e225.

PART VI

LABOR ANALGESIA

38

Neuraxial Labor Analgesia

Lindsay K. Sween, MD, MPH

BACKGROUND

Neuraxial analgesia is the most effective modality for pain control during labor and delivery and is used in ~70% of laboring women in the United States.[1,2] Compared to other pharmacologic and nonpharmacologic analgesic modalities, neuraxial analgesia provides better pain relief during the first and second stages of labor, improves patient attentiveness and cooperation, offers anesthesia for assisted vaginal delivery or cesarean delivery if necessary, and avoids the potentially negative maternal and neonatal respiratory effects of systemic opioid administration.[3] Over the past several decades, neuraxial options for labor analgesia have expanded from the standard epidural to include combined spinal epidural (CSE) and dural puncture epidural (DPE).

NEURAXIAL PROCEDURES

Neuraxial procedures for labor are typically placed in the L3-4, L4-5, or L5-S1 interspace.[3] The epidural space is commonly identified using the loss of resistance technique, a catheter is threaded into the space to allow for longer-term analgesia. If a CSE or DPE technique will be used, a small gauge spinal needle (usually 25-27 G) is inserted through the epidural needle ("needle-thru-needle" technique) until a "pop" is felt, and cerebrospinal fluid returns through the spinal needle. If spinal medication is desired, a small dose of local anesthetic medication (e.g., bupivacaine or ropivacaine) usually combined with a small dose of opioid (e.g., fentanyl or sufentanil) is injected into the intrathecal space. Then the spinal needle is removed, and a catheter is threaded into the epidural space to allow for longer-term analgesia.[1] A test dose should be administered to ensure that the epidural catheter is not intravenous or intrathecal. If no spinal medication was injected, the epidural catheter should be induced with a bolus of medication. We use 15 mL of the Beth Israel Deaconess standard solution (0.04% bupivacaine, fentanyl 1.67 µg/mL, epinephrine 1.67 µg/mL).

MAINTENANCE OF ANALGESIA

There are several techniques used to provide epidural analgesia. Continuous epidural infusion (CEI) using a set rate on an infusion pump allows for stable analgesia. When using the CEI technique, clinician bolus doses are administered when necessary to improve labor analgesia, or to provide additional analgesia for episiotomy, assisted vaginal delivery, repair of perineal tears after delivery, or to provide anesthesia for cesarean delivery.[3]

Patient-controlled epidural analgesia (PCEA) involves a patient self-administering preprogrammed boluses from an automated pump. This technique yields lower total local anesthetic dose, reduced number of clinician boluses, and decreased motor block compared to CEI.[1,3]

Some studies also suggest higher patient satisfaction, possibly due to increased perceived control over the analgesic process.[1,3] The PCEA technique can be combined with CEI, in which a patient receives a basal infusion and can be given additional self-administered boluses with a set lockout interval.[1,3] This combined CEI-PCEA technique provides improved analgesia and fewer clinician boluses compared to PCEA alone, although higher total doses of local anesthetic are administered.[1]

Programmed intermittent epidural boluses (PIEB) consists of an automated pump that delivers local anesthetic boluses at set intervals. Rapidly administered boluses yield increased dermatomal spread in the epidural space compared to the same volume infused slowly.[1] PIEB can be combined with PCEA, which has been shown to reduce local anesthetic requirements, increase patient satisfaction, and decrease the need for clinician-administered rescue boluses compared to CEI with PCEA.[4] One infrequently used technique is intermittent manual boluses, in which a clinician (anesthesiologist, midwife, or obstetrician) hand-boluses the epidural catheter with local anesthetic medication whenever the patient starts experiencing pain. This technique is labor intensive for the healthcare provider and may result in intervals of analgesia oscillating with periods of pain.[3]

INDICATIONS

- Per American College of Obstetricians and Gynecologists (ACOG), "In the absence of a medical contraindication, maternal request is a sufficient medical indication for pain relief during labor."[5]
- Although historically epidural analgesia was not used until at least 4 cm cervical dilation, multiple recent clinical trials have demonstrated that early epidural placement (at ≥1 cm dilation) does not increase the duration of labor or the rate of cesarean delivery.[6,7]
- Consider early placement for[3,8]:
  ○ Patients at risk for difficult placement (e.g., scoliosis, obesity).
  ○ Patients with potentially difficult airway to avoid the need for general anesthesia in the event of emergent cesarean delivery.
  ○ Patients with history of obstructive cardiac disease, in whom tachycardia and sudden decrease in systemic vascular resistance would be poorly tolerated (e.g., aortic stenosis, mitral stenosis, hypertrophic obstructive cardiomyopathy).
  ○ Patients with history of tachyarrhythmias (e.g., atrial fibrillation, supraventricular tachycardia).
  ○ Patients with concerning (e.g., category 2) fetal heart rate tracing, in whom emergent cesarean delivery may become necessary.
  ○ Patients with severe preeclampsia, especially if platelet count is trending down.
    ▪ Epidural analgesia may improve fetal perfusion in severe preeclampsia.

CONTRAINDICATIONS[3,5,8]

- Absolute contraindications:
  ○ Patient's refusal of neuraxial analgesia
  ○ Coagulopathy (e.g., coagulation factor deficiency, consumption, maternal hemorrhage, anticoagulant therapy)
  ○ Uncorrected hypovolemia
  ○ Skin or soft tissue infection at the site of intended epidural placement
  ○ Lack of resuscitative equipment or monitors

• Relative contraindications:
  ○ Thrombocytopenia and/or abnormal platelet function (congenital or acquired)
  ○ Untreated bacteremia
  ○ Space-occupying intracranial lesion with associated increased intracranial pressure

ADVANTAGES[8-10]

Advantages of the epidural technique:
• Continuous analgesia for prolonged periods of time
• Ability to provide anesthesia for cesarean delivery
• Immediate confirmation that epidural catheter is functional
• If a lower concentration local anesthetic solution is used at a higher infusion rate, there is a lower incidence of motor block and better dermatomal epidural spread resulting in a more consistent quality of analgesia

Advantages of the CSE technique:
• More rapid onset of analgesia compared to traditional epidural (mean difference 2.87 minutes; 95% CI 0.67-5.07)
• Improved analgesia with decreased need for supplemental bolus doses
• Fewer unilateral blocks and lower rate of epidural catheter failure (7-10% failure rate with CSE vs. 12-14% with standard epidural)
• Lower rate of epidural catheter replacement after CSE compared to standard epidural (3.2% with CSE compared to 7.1% with epidural)
• Higher patient satisfaction with analgesia from CSE compared to traditional epidural

DISADVANTAGES[8,11-13]

Disadvantages of epidural technique:
• Relatively slow onset of analgesia
• Larger medication doses required to attain effective analgesia when compared to spinal techniques (i.e., greater risk for maternal local anesthetic systemic toxicity)

Disadvantages of the CSE technique:
• Increased incidence of pruritus after CSE compared to standard epidural
• Possible higher risk for transient fetal bradycardia (proposed mechanism may be uterine tachysystole due to reduction of uterine β_2-adrenergic stimulation following a sudden decrease in circulating epinephrine with the rapid onset of analgesia after CSE [RR 1.31, 95% CI 1.02-1.67])
  ○ Can usually be treated with tocolytics and maternal blood pressure management and does not increase rate of cesarean delivery or worsen neonatal outcomes
• Spinal dose containing both local anesthetic and opioid may increase the incidence of hypotension, which would be poorly tolerated in patients with obstructive cardiac disease (e.g., stenotic heart lesions or hypertrophic obstructive cardiomyopathy)
• Theoretical risk for delayed recognition of epidural catheter failure (although this has not been seen in clinical trials, likely due to reduced catheter failure rate after CSE)

POTENTIAL SIDE EFFECTS[3,8,10,11]

- Hypotension (<10%, concentration dependent)
- Motor block (concentration dependent)
- Pruritus
- Shivering
- Urinary retention
- Accidental dural puncture with large bore needle (~1.5%)
- Postdural puncture headache (~1%)
- Inadequate analgesia (catheter replacement rate ~5%)
- Unintentional intravascular injection of local anesthetic medications (0.02%, 1:5,000)
- Unintentional intrathecal injection of local anesthetic medications (0.035%, 1:2900)
- High neuraxial blockade and total spinal anesthesia (0.006%, 1:16,200)
- Local tenderness at the site of epidural placement
- Nerve root injury from needle trauma
- Epidural abscess (0.2-3.7 in 100,000)
- Meningitis (0-3.5 in 100,000)
- Epidural hematoma (1 in 168,000)
- Transient fetal bradycardia

References

1. Nanji JA, Carvalho B. Modern techniques to optimize neuraxial labor analgesia. *Anesth Pain Med*. 2018;13:233-240.
2. Anim-Somuah M, Smyth RMD, Cyna AM, Cuthbert A. Epidural versus non-epidural or no analgesia for pain management in labour. *Cochrane Database of Systematic Reviews*. 2018;5:1-149.
3. Satpathy HK, Fleming AD, McGonigal ET, Barsoom MJ. Labor and delivery, analgesia, regional and local. Medscape. https://emedicine.medscape.com/article/149337-overview#showall. Updated July 29, 2020.
4. Wong CA, Ratliff JT, Sullivan JT, Scavone BM, Toledo P, McCarthy RJ. A randomized comparison of programmed intermittent epidural bolus with continuous epidural infusion for labor analgesia. *Anesth Analg*. 2006;102:904-909.
5. American College of Obstetricians and Gynecologists' Committee on Practice Bulletins—Obstetrics. ACOG Practice Bulletin No. 209: Obstetric analgesia and anesthesia. *Obstet Gynecol*. 2019;133(3):e208-e225.
6. Wong CA, Scavone BM, Peaceman AM, et al. The risk of cesarean delivery with neuraxial analgesia given early versus late in labor. *N Engl J Med*. 2005;352:655-665.
7. Wang FZ, Shen XF, Guo XR, Peng YZ, Gu XQ. Epidural analgesia in the latent phase of labor and the risk of cesarean delivery. *Anesthesiology*. 2009;111:871-880.
8. Wong CA. Epidural and spinal analgesia: anesthesia for labor and vaginal delivery. In: *Chestnut's Obstetric Anesthesia Principles and Practice*. 6th ed. Philadelphia, PA: Elsevier; 2020:474-539.
9. Sultan P, Murphy C, Halpern S, Carvalho B. The effect of low concentrations versus high concentrations of local anesthetics for labour analgesia on obstetric and anesthetic outcomes: a meta-analysis. *Can J Anesth*. 2013;60:840-854.
10. Silva M, Halpern SH. Epidural analgesia for labor: current techniques. *Local and Regional Anesthesia*. 2010;3:143-153.
11. Pan PH, Bogard TD, Owen MD. Incidence and characteristics of failures in obstetric neuraxial analgesia and anesthesia: a retrospective analysis of 19,259 deliveries. *Int J Obstet Anesth*. 2004;13:227-233.
12. Booth JM, Pan JC, Ross VH, Russell GB, Harris LC, Pan PH. Combined spinal epidural technique for labor analgesia does not delay recognition of epidural catheter failures: a single-center retrospective cohort survival analysis. *Anesthesiology*. 2016;125:516-524.
13. Cappiello E, O'Rourke N, Segal S, Tsen LC. A randomized trial of dural puncture epidural technique compared with the standard epidural technique for labor analgesia. *Anesth Analg*. 2008;107:1646-1651.

39

Low-Concentration Labor Epidural Analgesia

Lindsay K. Sween, MD, MPH

BACKGROUND

Of the pharmacologic and nonpharmacologic options for labor analgesia, neuraxial analgesia is the gold standard with the highest efficacy in terms of visual analog scale pain scores and patient satisfaction.[1] Historically, high concentration local anesthetic solutions (0.25-0.5% bupivacaine) were used to induce and maintain epidural analgesia. However, these epidural solutions resulted in significant hypotension, fetal bradycardia, maternal lower extremity motor blockade, and subsequent impaired second stage of labor.[1] More recently, dilute local anesthetic solutions (≤0.1% bupivacaine or equipotent ropivacaine) have gained favor due to decreased maternal motor block, increased maternal mobility, shorter second stage of labor, and decreased need for assisted vaginal delivery compared to more concentrated solutions.[1,2] Dilute local anesthetic solutions have been demonstrated to yield the same length of labor and rate of assisted vaginal delivery and cesarean delivery as nonepidural analgesic options.[3] Maternal satisfaction with labor analgesia has been shown to be equivalent with lower concentration epidural solutions compared to more concentrated solutions.[2,4]

GOALS

- To provide adequate labor analgesia while minimizing side effects (e.g., maternal motor block, hypotension, nausea/vomiting, pruritus, prolonged second stage of labor, need for assisted vaginal delivery, and fetal distress)

CLINICAL PRACTICE

Larger volumes of dilute local anesthetic solutions can safely be administered than of more concentrated solutions, which leads to enhanced analgesia via improved dermatomal spread in the epidural space.[1] The addition of a lipophilic opioid (e.g., fentanyl or sufentanil) to a dilute local anesthetic solution maximizes labor analgesia while reducing the required local anesthetic concentration.[1] Fentanyl and sufentanil have similar analgesic efficacy when administered in equipotent doses. Methods of administration include continuous epidural infusion of a fixed rate and a programmed intermittent epidural bolus (PIEB) in which a set volume is delivered by pump followed by a programmed pause. Both methods should be accompanied by a patient-controlled demand function (PCEA) to reduce the frequency of breakthrough pain.

The *"Walking Epidural"* solution from our tertiary care academic medical center is provided in Table 39-1.[5] This solution has been in continuous practice since the early 1990s. Table 39-2 lists variations of low-concentration to high-concentration (0.125%) schemes in common practice.

TABLE 39-1 • Recipes for Labor Epidural Analgesia at Beth Israel Deaconess Medical Center		
	Contents	**Notes**

Labor epidural solution	• BEF solution
	  ∘ Bupivacaine 0.04%
	  ∘ Fentanyl 1.67 µg/mL
	  ∘ May add 0.25 mL (250 µg) of epinephrine to 150 mL bag (1.67 mcg/mL)
		• After negative test dose, bolus 10-15 mL of BEF solution, then run at 15 mL/h

Labor epidural bolus	• 10 mL of BEF bolus off the pump **OR** • 8 mL of 0.125% bupivacaine (10 mg) + 2 mL of fentanyl (100 µg)	• Limit fentanyl to 100 µg/h

Note: For breakthrough pain, please refer to Chapter 42, "Refractory Pain During Labor Epidural Analgesia."
BEF, solution containing bupivacaine, epinephrine, and fentanyl.

TABLE 39-2 • Labor Epidural Solutions in Common Practice, Varying from Low to High Concentration				
Bupivacaine Concentration	**Adjuvant**	**Continuous Rate (mL/h)**	**PCEA Demand Dose (mL)**	**PIEB Setting**
0.04%	Fentanyl 1.7 µg/mL epinephrine 1.7 µg/mL	15	10	10 mL q40 min
0.063%	Fentanyl 2 µg/mL	12	8	8-10 mL q40 min
0.08%	Fentanyl 2 µg/mL	10	6	6-8 mL q40 min
0.10%	Fentanyl 2 µg/mL	8	5	6 mL q40 min
0.13%	Fentanyl 2-3 µg/mL	6	4	4-5 mL q40 min

PCEA, patient-controlled epidural analgesia; PIEB, programmed intermittent epidural analgesia.

SIDE EFFECTS

Compared to higher concentration local anesthetic solutions, dilute solutions are associated with a lower rate of assisted vaginal delivery, no change in the cesarean delivery rate, reduced incidence and severity of motor block, less urinary retention, and a shorter duration of the second stage of labor.[2] Higher and lower concentrations local anesthetic solutions produce similar rates of hypotension, maternal nausea and vomiting, fetal heart rate depression, and neonatal resuscitation.[2] One meta-analysis found an increased incidence of 1-minute Apgar scores <7 with high concentration epidural solutions but similar 5-minute Apgar scores between the high and low concentration groups.[2] Due to the addition of a lipophilic opioid, dilute local anesthetic solutions have a higher incidence of pruritus.[2]

Of note, the dose administered is similar among solutions; however, the low-concentration/high-volume solutions rely on the improvement in **distribution and dural surface area for diffusion**.

References

1. Nanji JA, Carvalho B. Modern techniques to optimize neuraxial labor analgesia. *Anesth Pain Med*. 2018;13:233-240.

2. Sultan P, Murphy C, Halpern S, Carvalho B. The effect of low concentrations versus high concentrations of local anesthetics for labour analgesia on obstetric and anesthetic outcomes: a meta-analysis. *Can J Anaesth*. 2013;60:840-854.

3. Wang TT, Sun S, Huang SQ. Effects of epidural labor analgesia with low concentrations of local anesthetics on obstetric outcomes: a systematic review and meta-analysis of randomized controlled trials. *Anesth Analg*. 2017;124:1571-1580.

4. Chestnut DH, Owen CI, Bates JN, Ostman LG, Choi WW, Geiger MW. Continuous infusion epidural analgesia during labor: a randomized, double-blind comparison of 0.0625% bupivacaine/0.0002% fentanyl versus 0.125% bupivacaine. *Anesthesiology*. 1988;68:754-759.

5. Breen TW, Shapiro T, Glass B, Foster-Payne D, Oriol NE. Epidural anesthesia for labor in an ambulatory patient. *Anesth Analg*. 1993;77:919-924.

40

Test Dose

Lindsay K. Sween, MD, MPH

BACKGROUND

Any and every injection into a presumed epidural catheter may unexpectedly be administered intravascularly or intrathecally. Local anesthetic should always be administered incrementally with aspiration before each dose![1]

Every Dose Is A Test Dose. Intravascular injection of local anesthetics can produce local anesthetic systemic toxicity (LAST)—a life-threatening condition that may result in seizures, cardiac arrhythmias, and cardiovascular collapse (Chapter 61, "Local Anesthetic Systemic Toxicity").[1] Inadvertent intrathecal injection of large doses of local anesthetics can lead to a high or total spinal anesthesia, which presents as paralysis, loss of consciousness, respiratory arrest, hypotension, bradycardia, and possible cardiac arrest (Chapter 60, "High Spinal").[2] The purpose of the test dose is to identify intravascular or intrathecal catheters using a small, safe dose of epinephrine-containing local anesthetic in order to prevent the consequences of a larger dose in the intravascular or intrathecal injection.[3] The classic test dose containing 3 mL of 1.5% lidocaine (45 mg) with 1:200,000 epinephrine (15 µg) was introduced by Moore and Batra in 1981.[4]

GOALS

- To identify intravascular and intrathecal catheters
- To prevent serious side effects
- To minimize false-positive results that lead to unnecessary catheter replacement

CLINICAL PRACTICE

The incidence of unintended intravascular catheter in the obstetric population is 4.9% to 7% with a stiff plastic epidural catheter but may be as low as <1% with a soft, flexible epidural catheter.[3,5] The incidence of intravascular injection undetected by aspiration is as high as 25% for single-orifice catheters and about 5% for multiorifice catheters. The incidence of unintended intrathecal catheter is 0.6% to 1.6%.[3] The incidence of subarachnoid injection after negative aspiration is between 0.06% and 0.0008%.[3]

A positive test dose is defined as:

- Heart rate increase >10 beats per minute at 25 to 30 seconds after the injection of 10 or 15 µg epinephrine.
- Observation of both a metallic taste and tinnitus after the injection of at least 100 mg lidocaine.

- Warm or heavy sensation in the lower extremities at 3 minutes, or inability to raise legs at 4 to 10 minutes after injection of 30 or 45 mg lidocaine.[3]
- The sensitivity of a test dose is reduced in the parturient in labor or who is on β-blockers.

SIDE EFFECTS

The intravenous or epidural injection of epinephrine has the potential to cause vasoconstriction resulting in decreased uteroplacental blood flow, which may lead to fetal bradycardia.[6] If the epidural catheter is intravascular, intravenous injection of epinephrine may induce maternal tachyarrhythmias.[6] If the epidural catheter is intrathecal, total spinal block and respiratory paralysis are extremely rare but possible with the relatively low dose of lidocaine utilized for a test dose.[6,7] Subarachnoid injection of lidocaine may also produce sympathectomy and maternal hypotension leading to decreased uteroplacental perfusion and possible fetal bradycardia.[6,7]

CONTRAINDICATIONS

Epinephrine-containing test dose is contraindicated in patients with history of tachyarrhythmia (e.g., supraventricular tachycardia, atrial fibrillation, or Wolff–Parkinson–White syndrome) or in whom tachycardia would be poorly tolerated (e.g., obstructive cardiac disease). Similarly, lidocaine test dose is contraindicated in patients who would poorly tolerate sympathectomy and its resultant hypotension and tachycardia (e.g., aortic stenosis, mitral stenosis, or hypertrophic obstructive cardiomyopathy).[6]

References

1. El-Boghdadly K, Pawa A, Chin KJ. Local anesthetic systemic toxicity: current perspectives. *Local Reg Anesth.* 2018;11:35-44.
2. Liu H, Tariq R, Liu GL, Yan H, Kaye AD. Inadvertent intrathecal injections and best practice management. *Acta Anaesthesiologica Scandinavica.* 2017;61(1):11-22.
3. Guay J. The epidural test dose: A review. *Anesth Analg.* 2006;102:921-929.
4. Moore DC, Batra MS. The components of an effective test dose prior to epidural block. *Anesthesiology.* 1981;55:693-696.
5. Spiegel JE, Vasudevan A, Li Y, Hess PE. A randomized prospective study comparing two flexible epidural catheters for labour analgesia. *Br J Anaesth.* 2009;103(3):400-405.
6. Nathan N and Wong CA. Spinal, epidural, and caudal anesthesia: anatomy, physiology, and technique. In: Chestnut DH, Wong CA, Tsen LC, et al., eds. *Chestnut's Obstetric Anesthesia: Principles and Practice.* 6th ed. Philadelphia, PA: Elsevier. 2020; 238-270.
7. Pratt S, Vasudevan A, Hess P. A prospective randomized trial of lidocaine 30 mg versus 45 mg for epidural test dose for intrathecal injection in the obstetric population. *Anesth Analg.* 2013;116(1):125-132.

41

Epidural Morphine Following Vaginal Delivery

Merry I. Colella, MD

BACKGROUND

- Pain after vaginal delivery can interfere with a mother's daily activities and ability to care for her newborn.
- Acute postpartum pain may be particularly significant for women who have undergone an episiotomy or instrumented delivery, or who have experienced extended perineal tears or uterine involution.
- The use of epidural morphine for select parturients may help to improve pain control after vaginal delivery and reduce the need for oral opioids.[1,2]

PATIENT SELECTION

- Did the patient undergo any of the following?
  - Third- or fourth-degree perineal episiotomy or laceration.
  - Prolonged or complicated repair of episiotomy or laceration.
  - Instrumented delivery.
  - Uterine involution.
- Is the patient also complaining of significant pain prior to removal of epidural?
  - A common marker of above average pain is the need for an additional epidural bolus medication following or during the laceration repair.

  If **YES**:
- Discuss with the obstetric team and suggest epidural morphine.
- Explain the benefits and possible side effects to patient.
- Consider giving epidural morphine prior to removal of the labor epidural catheter.

CLINICAL PRACTICE

If administration of epidural morphine is desired, the protocol at Beth Israel Deaconess Medical Center is as follows (Chapter 54, "Neuraxial Morphine"):
- Give 1.5 to 2 mg epidural morphine.

- Document the administration dose, time, and route in the online medical record, as the patient will need to be closely monitored for respiratory depression for 18 hours following administration.
  - Include orders for ketorolac, acetaminophen, naloxone bolus, naloxone drip, and antiemetics as provided in the obstetric anesthesia neuraxial morphine order set.
- Hand the neuraxial morphine monitoring form to the nurse and be sure to fill out:
  - Date and time of morphine administration.
  - Date, time, and mode of delivery.
- Give appropriate sign-out to the obstetric team and the nurse.
- The labor and delivery nurse should communicate about the administration of neuraxial morphine with postpartum nursing.
- Alert the obstetric anesthesia team and give sign-out to the oncoming call team.
- Remember: No additional narcotics or sedatives should then be given to the patient for the following 24 hours.

References

1. Goodman SR, Drachenberg AM, Johnson SA, et al. Decreased postpartum use of oral pain medication after a single dose of epidural morphine. *Reg Anesth Pain Med*. 2005;30:134-139.
2. Macarthur A, Imarengiaye C, Tureanu L, et al. A randomized, double-blind, placebo-controlled trial of epidural morphine analgesia after vaginal delivery. *Anesth Analg*. 2010;110(1):159-164.

42

Refractory Pain During Labor Epidural Analgesia

Erin J. Ciampa, MD, PhD
Philip E. Hess, MD

BACKGROUND

The majority of patients achieve effective relief of labor pain with a standard infusion of a low-concentration local anesthetic and opioid mixture with a patient-controlled bolus option; however, some patients present with refractory pain. Determining the underlying reason for refractory pain is critical to guide effective treatment, and most cases can be resolved with appropriate intervention.

Refractory pain can be a sign of dysfunctional labor. Inherently in this subset of patient population, they have increased incidence of intrapartum cesarean delivery.[1] Prompt management of refractory pain is important to improve maternal satisfaction and ensure the successful conversion of labor epidural analgesia to anesthesia for subsequent cesarean section.

GOALS

- To provide a framework for determining the etiology of refractory pain in a patient receiving labor epidural analgesia
- To describe interventions corresponding to each root factor underlying refractory pain

COMMON CAUSES OF REFRACTORY PAIN AND GUIDED INTERVENTIONS

There are two major categories of scenario in which refractory labor pain occurs: epidural catheter failure versus analgesia failure.

Catheter Failure

It is characterized by **failure to achieve or maintain a bilateral sensory block**. The catheter may provide effective analgesia after a bolus, but regresses to an inadequate level between boluses. This is usually because the infusion is not targeting the epidural space due to one of the scenarios listed in Table 42-1.

Analgesia Failure

It is characterized by presence of refractory pain **despite bilateral sensory block**. Refractory pain in the setting of a functioning epidural that generates bilateral sensory block can be due to any of the scenarios listed in Table 42-2.

TABLE 42-1 • Causes and Treatments of Epidural Catheter Failure

Underlying Reason	Clinical Findings	Remedy
Catheter was mis-sited, e.g., to paravertebral space or catheter pointed to sacral direction	Asymmetric block, may appear bilateral after boluses, but persists as asymmetric and at low levels	Replace epidural
Catheter has migrated	No sensory level or receding sensory level Catheter depth from skin may be less than distance at time of placement	Replace epidural
Epidural infusion interrupted	No sensory level or receding sensory level due to pump malfunction or disconnection at catheter/filter/tubing junctions	Check the epidural pump Clean and reconnect sterilely Administer bolus to reinitiate epidural analgesia Replace tubing set if hourly volume not achieved

TABLE 42-2 • Causes and Treatments of Labor Analgesia Failure

Underlying Reasons	Clinical Findings	Remedy
Inadequate volume	Sensory block does not reach T10	Raise level with *volume* Provide bolus, favoring volume over local anesthetic concentration (e.g., bolus off the pump)
Inadequate block density	Adequate sensory level bilaterally but patient reports breakthrough pain	Make block *denser* Provide bolus, favoring local anesthetic concentration over volume (e.g., 8 mL of 0.125% bupivacaine ± 100 µg fentanyl)
Pain coming from sources other than uterine contractions (e.g., full bladder, uterine rupture, liver hematoma, amniotic fluid embolism, chorioamnionitis)	Varied depending on clinical scenario, but heralds include constant pain, chest pain, non-reassuring fetal status, maternal vital sign instability	Interrogate pain characteristics (Remits between contractions? Sharp versus dull? Radiating versus localized?) and other clinical signs Pursue diagnostic tests in consultation with obstetric team to determine cause of pain and appropriate care
Dysfunctional labor with secondary hyperalgesia Breakthrough pain algorithm (Fig. 42-1)	Refractory pain despite adequate sensory block and administration of dense local anesthetic boluses +/− Slow or stalled labor progress	Consider increasing concentration of epidural solution from 0.04% to 0.125% bupivacaine (see "Preparation of 0.125% Bupivacaine Infusion Solution"), run at 10-12 mL/h, patient controlled epidural analgesia bolus dose 0 to 5 mL q20 min Consider new CSE—dense block from new labor spinal will usually provide temporary relief Consider other adjuncts given epidurally (bolus 10-20 µg dexmedetomidine,[2] or infusion at 0.5 µg/mL) or spinal morphine (100 µg)[3]

(Continued)

TABLE 42-2 • Causes and Treatments of Labor Analgesia Failure (*Continued*)		
Underlying Reasons	**Clinical Findings**	**Remedy**
Fetal malposition	Constant back pain between the shoulder blades and/or neck pain unrelated to uterine contraction despite adequate sensory block	The mechanism is poorly understood; usually, it occurs in the situation with fetal occiput posterior or occiput transverse position, which may affect epidural compliance Concentrate epidural solution (e.g., 0.125% bupivacaine with fentanyl 5 μg/mL ± dexmedetomidine 1 μg/mL at 5 mL/h) to decrease volume ± pause epidural infusion for 1 hour

Preparation of 0.125% Bupivacaine Infusion Solution

0.25% Bupivacaine	30 mL
Normal Saline, preservative free	26 mL
Fentanyl (50 μg/mL ampule)	4 mL (200 μg)
Total volume = 60 mL of 0.125% bupivacaine with 3.3 μg/mL fentanyl	

BREAKTHROUGH PAIN ALGORITHM (FIG. 42-1)

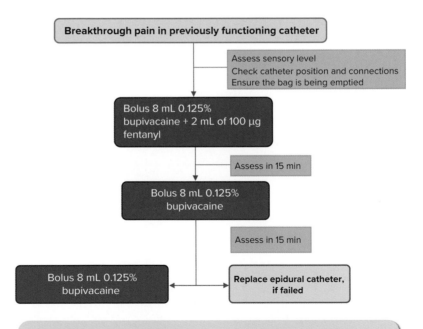

FIGURE 42-1 • Breakthrough pain algorithm.

References

1. Hess PE, Pratt SD, Soni AK, et al. An association between severe labor pain and cesarean delivery. *Anesth Analg.* 2000;90:881-886.

2. Zhao Y, Xin Y, Liu Y, Yi X, Liu Y. Effect of epidural dexmedetomidine combined with ropivacaine in labor analgesia: a randomized double-blinded controlled study. *Clin J Pain.* 2017;33(4):319-324.

3. Vasudevan A, Snowman CE, Sundar S, Sarge TW, Hess PE. Intrathecal morphine reduces breakthrough pain during labour epidural analgesia. *Br J Anaesth.* 2007;98(2):241-245.

43

Pruritus from Labor Analgesia

John J. Kowalczyk, MD

BACKGROUND AND INITIAL EVALUATION

- Pruritus is a side effect of neuraxial opioids.
- Evaluate the patient and assess the relative degree of itching.
- Itching is an expected side effect that is often mild and may be self-limiting if associated with spinal fentanyl for labor. Approximately an hour and a half after the spinal dose for labor, itching improves in the majority of patients.
- The majority of patients do not need medications to treat pruritus. An explanation and reassurance are often sufficient until the spinal dose of fentanyl no longer has an effect.
- Only if itching is significantly bothersome to the patient should a treatment option be offered.
- Treatment with antagonists and agonist-antagonist could intrinsically reverse the labor analgesia. Use with caution.

OMISSION OF NEURAXIAL OPIOID—FIRST CHOICE

- For patients with severe itching during labor or prior history of unremitting, severe itching, opioids may be omitted from labor epidural infusion or neuraxial morphine from cesarean analgesia.
- For labor, fentanyl has been shown to reduce the necessary local anesthetics dose by 25% to 40%. Omission of fentanyl usually requires an increase in bupivacaine concentration to 0.125% for the labor epidural.
  - It has been this author's experience that the vast majority of patients who request a switch to an opioid-free epidural solution ultimately request to be changed back, either due to increased pain or increased sensory and motor blockade. Careful counseling and exhaustion of the above options are essential before making this switch.
  - Replace fentanyl with 0.5 µg/mL dexmedetomidine (with bupivacaine) for labor epidural (Chapter 6, "Dexmedetomidine").
- Increased pain should be expected and may necessitate higher local anesthetic concentration infusion or alternative epidural adjuncts for labor or additional post-cesarean pain relief treatment options.

TREATMENT OPTIONS—SECOND CHOICE

Caution to use nalbuphine or naloxone for the laboring patients who may undergo intrapartum cesarean delivery or for who is during cesarean surgery. It may cause refractory pain after cesarean section.

- Nalbuphine[1-3]:
  - Dose: 2.5 mg IV/IM, may repeat two times.
  - Shown to be more effective than placebo, diphenhydramine, propofol, or naloxone.
  - May also improve opioid-induced nausea/vomiting and respiratory depression.
  - However, it can cause sedation at higher doses.
  - Four or more doses have been shown to decrease the effectiveness of neuraxial opioids.
- Naloxone:
  - Found to be less effective than nalbuphine.
  - Dose: 40 to 80 µg IV, may repeat three times or utilize infusion.
  - As an opioid-antagonist, it will also improve opioid-induced nausea/vomiting and respiratory depression.
  - Does not cause sedation.
  - However, can cause increased pain scores at higher doses.

DIPHENHYDRAMINE

- This should **NOT** be considered a treatment if the itching is thought to be caused by a neuraxial (spinal or epidural) opioid.
- Opioid-induced histamine release from mast cells is not the mechanism for pruritus after neuraxial opioid administration.
- Studies have shown limited success when compared to placebo and markedly reduced effect when compared to nalbuphine.

References

1. Cohen SE, Rantner EF, Kreitzman TR, et al. Nalbuphine is better than naloxone for treatment of side effects after epidural morphine. *Anesth Analg.* 1992;75(5):747-752.
2. Somrat C, Oranuch K, Ketchada U, et al. Optimal dose of nalbuphine for treatment of intrathecal-morphine induced pruritus after caesarean section. *J Obstet Gynaecol Res.* 1999;25(3):209-213.
3. Jannuzzi RG. Nalbuphine for treatment of opioid-induced pruritus: a systematic review of literature. *Clin J Pain.* 2016;32(1):87-93.

44

Intravenous Analgesia

Lindsay K. Sween, MD, MPH

BACKGROUND

Intravenous patient-controlled analgesia (PCA) with fentanyl or remifentanil is an option for labor analgesia in patients for whom neuraxial anesthesia is contraindicated (e.g., platelet disorders, coagulopathy, or patient's refusal).[1] Both remifentanil and fentanyl PCA have significantly lower visual analog scale pain scores 1 hour after treatment initiation compared to baseline, with pain score reduction being significantly greater with remifentanil compared to fentanyl.[1,2] Patients' pain scores with fentanyl and remifentanil PCA return to baseline by 3 hours after treatment initiation, likely reflecting increased pain levels with advancing labor.[1]

METHOD OF ADMINISTRATION

Fentanyl

A starting dose for fentanyl intravenous PCA is 12.5 µg with a lockout interval of 6 minutes and can be increased to 25 µg every 6 minutes, if needed. Maximum hourly dose is 250 µg.[1,3] To minimize maternal and fetal opioid exposure and related side effects, there should not be a basal infusion rate.[1,3] Fentanyl has a rapid onset of action, because its high lipophilicity permits rapid distribution from plasma into highly vascularized compartments, muscle, and fat. The transfer half-life into the central nervous system is 4.7 to 6.6 minutes.[4] Fentanyl is metabolized by the $3A_4$ substrate of the CYP450 system in the liver with an elimination half-life of 3 to 8 hours.[4]

Remifentanil

The intravenous PCA dose of remifentanil for labor analgesia is 0.2 to 0.8 µg/kg (with an increment of 0.1 µg/kg) with a lockout interval of 2 to 3 minutes.[5] Remifentanil has a more rapid onset of action than fentanyl with onset within 1 minute and peak effect in 2 minutes.[6] Remifentanil is rapidly hydrolyzed by plasma esterase leading to a context-sensitive half-life of 3 to 4 minutes and an elimination half-time of 10 to 20 minutes.[1]

SIDE EFFECTS

With both fentanyl and remifentanil PCA, patient-reported pain scores are significantly higher and patient satisfaction is lower than with neuraxial epidural analgesia.[2] Both remifentanil and fentanyl are associated with maternal respiratory depression and episodic desaturation (oxygen saturation <95%), and thus necessitate continuous patient monitoring with respiratory rate and pulse oximetry.[1,5,6] Remifentanil is associated with significantly increased maternal sedation compared to fentanyl or epidural analgesia.[1,5,6] Remifentanil also has a greater incidence of pruritus than fentanyl.[1]

Reduced fetal heart rate beat-to-beat variability has been associated with remifentanil.[5] However, remifentanil is not associated with an increased rate of newborns having Apgar scores less than 7 at 5 minutes compared to epidural analgesia.[2] There is no significant difference in Apgar scores or umbilical cord blood gas in babies born to mothers who received fentanyl or remifentanil when they are compared to each other or to epidural analgesia.[1,2,7] The rate of cesarean delivery is similar in mothers using fentanyl, remifentanil, and epidural labor analgesia.[1,2]

References

1. Douma MR, Verwey RA, Kam-Endtz CE, van der Linden PD, Stienstra R. Obstetric analgesia: a comparison of patient-controlled meperidine, remifentanil, and fentanyl in labour. *Br J Anaesth*. 2010;104(2):209-215.

2. Weibel S, Jelting Y, Afshari A, et al. Patient-controlled analgesia with remifentanil versus alternative parenteral methods for pain management in labour. *Cochrane Database Syst Rev*. 2017;4(4):CD011989.

3. Hosokawa Y, Morisaki H, Nakatsuka I, et al. Retrospective evaluation of intravenous fentanyl patient-controlled analgesia during labor. *J Anaesth*. 2012;26:219-224.

4. Schug SA, Ting S. Fentanyl formulations in the management of pain: an update. *Drugs*. 2017;77:747-763.

5. Volmanen P, Akural EI, Raudaskoski T, Alahuhta S. Remifentanil in obstetric analgesia: a dose-finding study. *Anesth Analg*. 2002;94(4):913-917.

6. Devabhakthuni S. Efficacy and safety of remifentanil as an alternative labor analgesic. *Clin Med Insights Women's Health*. 2013;6:37-49.

7. Nikkola EM, Ekblad UU, Kero PO, Alihanka JJM, Salonen MAO. Intravenous fentanyl PCA during labour. *Can J Anaesth*. 1997;44(12):1248-1255.

45

Operative Vaginal Delivery

Galina V. Korsunsky, MD

BACKGROUND

Operative vaginal delivery (VD) remains an essential component of labor management, accounting for 3% to 6% of all deliveries, and includes forceps and vacuum-assisted births. Operative VD is used to expedite safe VD for maternal and/or fetal indications.[1,2]

- Maternal indications:
  - Maternal exhaustion
  - Ineffective pushing in the second stage of labor
  - Need to avoid pushing in the second stage due to maternal cardiac or neurologic disease
  - Prolonged second stage
- Fetal indications:
  - Non-reassuring fetal heart rate during the second stage of labor

Operative VD can cause significant maternal and fetal morbidities.[3-5] These should be compared to cesarean delivery (CD) outcomes, and maternal and fetal complications should be considered for both prior to operative VD.

COMPLICATIONS

Maternal complications from operative VD include increased rates of the following:

- Third- and fourth-degree perineal tears
- Anal sphincter injury
- Fecal incontinence
- Vaginal and cervical lacerations
- Postpartum hemorrhage
- Urinary retention
- Urinary incontinence

Newborn complications from operative VD vary somewhat based on the device used. They include increased rates of the following:

- Scalp laceration
- Cephalohematoma
- Subgaleal hemorrhage[6]
- Cerebral hemorrhage
- Skull fracture

- Brachial plexus injury
- Facial nerve palsy
- Facial lacerations
- Corneal abrasions
- External ocular injury
- Retinal hemorrhage

CONTRAINDICATIONS

Specific criteria must be met prior to operative VD. This includes fetal vertex presentation, fully dilated cervix, known fetal head position, obstetrician's familiarity and experience with an instrument, and ability to perform an emergency CD if needed, to name a few.

Operative VD is contraindicated in the following instances:

- Fetal head is not engaged.
- The position of the head is not known.
- Fetus has a known or suspected bone demineralization condition.
- Fetus has a known or suspected bleeding disorder.

ANESTHETIC MANAGEMENT

In order to perform an operative VD, a parturient has to have adequate anesthesia. The anesthesiologist should be alerted and present, and should assess the epidural level and functional status prior to obstetricians initiating operative VD. We recommend a 5- to 10-mL bolus of 3% bicarbonated chloroprocaine epidurally to aid maternal comfort for operative VD without hampering maternal pushing effort. An anesthesia provider should stay with the patient to ensure adequate anesthesia and be ready for an emergent CD, anticipating and managing any subsequent postpartum hemorrhage.

References

1. ACOG practice bulletin. Operative vaginal delivery. *Obstet Gynecol*. 2020;135(4):e149-e159.
2. Ali UA, Notwitz ER. Vacuum assisted vaginal delivery. *Rev Obstet Gynecol*. 2009;2(1):5-17.
3. Salman L, Aviram A, Krispin E, Wiznitzer A, Chen R, Gabbay-Benziv R. Adverse neonatal and maternal outcome following vacuum-assisted vaginal delivery: does indication matter? *Arch Gynecol Obstet*. 2017;295:1145-1150.
4. Johnson JH, Figueroa R, Garry D, Elimian A, Maulik D. Immediate maternal and neonatal effects of forceps and vacuum-assisted deliveries. *Obstet Gynecol*. 2004;103(3):513-518.
5. Rottenstreich M, Rotem R, Katz B, Rottenstreich A, Grisaru-Granovsky S. Vacuum extraction delivery at first vaginal birth following cesarean: maternal and neonatal outcome. *Arch Gynecol Obstet*. 2020:301:483-489.
6. Levin G, Mankuta D, Eventov-Friedman S. Factors associated with the severity of neonatal subgaleal haemorrhage following vacuum assisted delivery. *Eur J Obstet Gynecol Reprod Biol*. 2020;245:205-209.

46

Twin Delivery

Yunping Li, MD

BACKGROUND

- The incidence of multifetal gestations has increased dramatically in the United States due to:
  - Advanced maternal age when multifetal gestations are more likely to occur naturally (Odds Ratio = 4.5) compared to younger women.
  - Increased use of assisted reproductive technology.[1]
- Major perinatal complications are increased with multiple gestations, including preterm birth, fetal anomalies, preeclampsia, and gestational diabetes. The risk of stillbirth begins to increase significantly at approximately 38 weeks of gestational age.
- Types of twin pregnancy include monochorionic/monoamniotic twins, monochorionic/diamniotic twins, and dichorionic/diamniotic twins.
- Based on standard obstetric nomenclature, Twin A is the presenting twin.
- The optimal route and timing of delivery in women with multifetal gestations depend on multiple factors, including the type of gestation, fetal presentations, fetal weight, gestational age, and the experience of the obstetricians.[1]
- Delivery timing: uncomplicated dichorionic twins 37 to 38 weeks gestation; uncomplicated monochorionic diamnionic twins 34 to 36 weeks gestation; uncomplicated monochorionic monoamniotic twins 32 to 34 weeks gestation.
- Vaginal delivery is a reasonable option.[2] However, monoamniotic twins are delivered by cesarean between 32 and 34 weeks of gestation to avoid an umbilical cord complication.
- Options for delivery of the second nonvertex presenting twin include:
  - Breech extraction.
  - Internal podalic version with breech extraction.
  - Internal cephalic version.
  - Cesarean delivery.
- Possible cesarean delivery could be called during twin delivery for one or both twins.

FOR ANESTHESIOLOGISTS

- As always, ensure that you have a functional epidural.
- All twin vaginal delivery should occur in the operating room. At the commencement of the second stage of labor, the patient should be moved to an operating room.
- For a multiparous woman, she may enter the operating room earlier in anticipation of rapid delivery.

- Close the anesthesia record in the labor room and continue the same record in the operating room.
- Assist the nurse with the transfer of the patient to an operating room so that the epidural pump and medications can be safely continued.
- Continue labor epidural infusion.
- An anesthesia resident and attending should be present for the delivery of twins.
- Be prepared for **emergent** cesarean delivery. Chloroprocaine 3% and bicarbonate should be available to draw and dose quickly.
- Emergencies are uncommon after the delivery of Twin A, but must be prepared for emergent cesarean delivery.
  - Twin B changes lie to transverse or breech.
  - Placental abruption with fetal heart rate (FHR) abnormality or bradycardia.
  - Twin B has cord prolapse.
  - Twin B's head engages the cervix/pelvis for the first time and experiences a prolonged FHR deceleration.
- The anesthesia team may step out once both babies are delivered and adequate uterine tone has been achieved. In some nulliparous women, it may take a significant amount of additional time to deliver Twin B, sometimes even leading to the mother returning to the labor room. If this is the intended plan, ensure that Twin B maintains a cephalic position and is stable for several contractions (>10-15 minutes).
- If magnesium sulfate is used for fetal neuroprotection, the infusion can be discontinued after delivery of Twin B. This may improve uterine tone and decrease the risk of postpartum hemorrhage.

References

1. American College of Obstetrics and Gynecology, Practice Bulletin No. 231. Multifetal gestations: twin, triplet and high-order multifetal pregnancies. *Obstet Gynecol*. 2021;137(6):e145-e162.
2. Barrett JFR, Hannah ME, Hutton EK, et al. A randomized trial of planned cesarean or vaginal delivery for twin pregnancy. *N Engl J Med*. 2013;369(14):1295-1305.

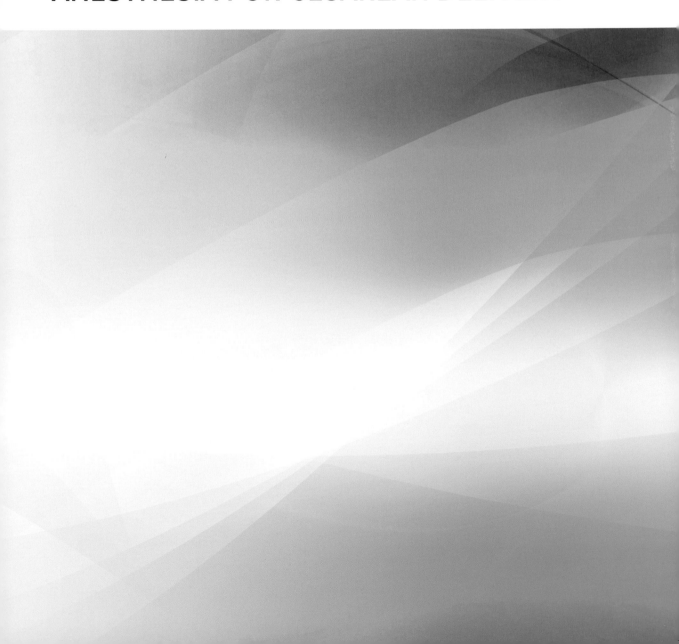

PART VII

ANESTHESIA FOR CESAREAN DELIVERY

47

Neuraxial Anesthesia for Cesarean Delivery

Philip E. Hess, MD

BACKGROUND

Cesarean delivery (CD) ranks among the most common surgical procedures in the world. Yet, too many women die during childbirth. Regional anesthesia had been used in obstetrics since 1940s.[1] Evolving knowledge and clinical advances in obstetric anesthesiology made significant contributions in the field of neuraxial anesthesia. Today, regional anesthesia is safer and more effective than ever because of countless contributions of researchers around the world.

Contributing factors to improving maternal satisfaction, patient safety, and decreases in anesthesia-related maternal mortality and morbidity in Obstetric Anesthesia include:

- Increased use of neuraxial anesthesia and decreased use of general anesthesia[2,3]
- High-quality and preservative-free (PF) medications
- Use of neuraxial morphine for long duration of postoperative analgesia
- Test dose for epidural catheters to identify intrathecal and intravascular catheter, and incremental dosing of epidural medications
- Advances in the design of epidural catheter
- Advances in the design of epidural and spinal needles to decrease the incidence of postdural puncture headache and nerve injury

ADVANTAGES OF NEURAXIAL ANESTHESIA FOR CESAREAN DELIVERY

- Avoid general anesthesia and potential difficult airway.
- Lower risk of aspiration.
- Less blood loss, possible due to lower mean blood pressure and lack of effect of uterine atony from inhalational agents.
- Minimal placental drug transfer.
- No inhalational agents needed and less pollution.
- Ability to install neuraxial morphine for much better postoperative analgesia.
- Awake mother is allowed to experience childbirth.

CONTRAINDICATIONS FOR NEURAXIAL ANESTHESIA

- Patient refusal
- Allergy to local anesthetics (true allergy to amides is extremely rare)
- Coagulopathy and severe thrombocytopenia
- Local infection at the insertion site
- Uncorrected hypovolemia
- Lack of monitoring or resuscitative equipment

  Relative contraindications:
- Increased intracranial pressure (avoid dural puncture)
- Uncooperative patient
- Obstructive cardiac lesion (avoid spinal anesthesia)
- Systemic or remote infection

POTENTIAL RISKS AND SIDE EFFECTS

- Failed spinal: Usually it is a technical failure; rarely it is because of anatomical variation[4,5]
- Failure conversion of labor epidural to epidural anesthesia for CD (Chapter 49, "Conversion of Labor Epidural for Cesarean Delivery")
- Postdural puncture headache (Chapter 64, "Postdural Puncture Headache)
- Severe nerve injury (Chapter 62, "Peripartum Neurological Complications")
- High spinal or total spinal (Chapter 60, "High Spinal")
- Hypotension (Chapter 50, "Hypotension After Spinal Anesthesia")
- Nausea, vomiting, and pruritus (Chapter 57, "Side Effects of Neuraxial Opioids")

CLINICAL POINTS

- Spinal injection should be below the L2 vertebra to avoid potential contact with the spinal cord. Ultrasound confirmation in patients with morbid obesity and/or scoliosis may be helpful.
- Aseptic technique is a must—always wear a mask and a cap for neuraxial procedures.
- Spinal injection is a **HIGH-RISK** procedure. Two sets of eyes should verify the medications before injection.
- A **T4** sensory blockage is appropriate for CD under neuraxial anesthesia. The sensory afferent nerves innervating the abdomen and pelvic organs accompany sympathetic trunk from L1 to T5. The neurotomes of C3-C5 provide innervation of the diaphragm and must be avoided.[6-8]
- Smaller doses of local anesthetic result in a lower blockage level (at T6 or lower) and have a lower incidence of hypotension, but at the cost of patient discomfort, especially with visceral stimulation.
- Assessment of sensory block by cold, pinprick, and touch can vary quite differently.[6,7] The pinprick method is encouraged as anesthesia—not analgesia—is required for surgery.
- The choice of neuraxial procedure should be based on the individual patient, considering the expected surgical time, patient comorbidities, and fetal factors. See the next section "Decision Making."

DECISION MAKING (TABLE 47-1)

TABLE 47-1 • Choice of Neuraxial Anesthetic for Cesarean Delivery		
Spinal Anesthesia • Expected ≤90 minutes • Primary or first repeat CD • Normal BMI	**CSE** • Possibly >90 minutes • Multiple repeat CD • Prior surgery • High BMI • Elevated bleeding risks: accreta, previa	**Epidural** • Expected >90 minutes • Multiple surgeries, surgical mesh • Slow and controllable sympathectomy, ideal for cardiac disease

BMI, body mass index; CD, cesarean delivery; CSE, combined spinal and epidural.

MEDICATION AND DOSAGE (BOX 47-1)

BOX 47-1 • The Standard Medications for Cesarean Delivery at Beth Israel Deaconess Medical Center

Spinal Medications
- 0.75% hyperbaric bupivacaine, 1.5 mL +/− 0.2 mL if ≤60 *or* ≥70 in   (11.25 mg)
- Fentanyl 0.5 mL   (25 µg)
- PF Morphine 0.3-0.5 mL   (150-250 µg)

Blood Pressure
- Phenylephrine, pre-med 10 mL syringe, if heart rate (HR) >90, give 100 µg
- Can also run a phenylephrine infusion at 0.5 µg/kg/min, titrate
- Ephedrine, pre-med 5 mL syringe, if HR <70, give 10 mg
- If HR 70 to 90, 5 mg ephedrine + 100 µg phenylephrine

Other Medications
- Antibiotics, prefer 2 g cefazolin; if body weight >110 kg, use 3 g
- Oxytocin 20 IU/1000 mL, set up at 250 mL/h for infusion
- Uterotonics (available in-room fridge)
- Oxygen via a face mask, if O_2 saturation <95%

References

1. Marx GF. Regional analgesia in obstetrics. *Anaesthesist*. 1972; 21(3):84-91.
2. Hawkins JL, Chang J, Palmer SK, Gibbs CP, Callaghan WM. Anesthesia-related maternal mortality in the United States: 1979-2002. *Obstet Gynecol*. 2011;117:69-74.
3. Lim G, Facco FL, Nathan N, et al. A review of the impact of obstetric anesthesia on maternal and neonatal outcomes. *Anesthesiology*. 2018;129(1):192-215.
4. Hoppe J, Popham P. Complete failure of spinal anaesthesia in obstetrics. *Int J Obstet Anesth*. 2007;16(3):250-255.
5. Spiegel JE, Hess PE. Large intrathecal volume: a cause of true failed spinal anesthesia. *J Anesth*. 2007;21(3):399-402.
6. Hoyle J, Yentis AM. Assessing the height of block for cesarean section over the past three decades: trends from the literature. *Anaesthesia*. 2015;70:421-428.
7. Russell IF. Levels of anaesthesia and intraoperative pain at caesarean section under regional block. *Int J Obstet Anesth*. 1995;4(2):71-77.
8. Tsen LC, Bateman BT. Anesthesia for cesarean delivery. In: *Chestnut's Obstetric Anesthesia Principles and Practice*. 6th ed. Philadelphia: Elsevier; 2020:568-626.

48

General Anesthesia for Cesarean Delivery

John J. Kowalczyk, MD

BACKGROUND

- General anesthesia (GA) has largely been replaced by neuraxial due to decreased maternal mortality and morbidity and improved fetal outcomes (Chapter 47, "Neuraxial Anesthesia for Cesarean Delivery").
- Indications:
  - Maternal refusal of neuraxial anesthesia.
  - Severe psychiatric or developmental disorder.
  - Coagulopathy.
  - Local infection at the neuraxial site.
  - Severe, uncorrected hypovolemia.
  - Intracranial mass with increased intracranial pressure.
  - Failure of the neuraxial block to rise in urgent or emergent cesarean.
  - Umbilical cord prolapse with persistent fetal bradycardia.
  - Incomplete coverage of spinal anesthesia.
  - Multiple failed neuraxial placements.
  - Persistent intraoperative pain that is uncontrolled.
- STAT or urgent intrapartum indications for GA should involve constant communication between the obstetrician and anesthesiologist. This ensures a continued need for GA and updates everyone on the current steps in the ongoing process.

PREOPERATIVE

- Perform standard evaluation, consent, and multidisciplinary huddle.
- Place a 16 or 18 G peripheral intravenous catheter and obtain a complete blood count and type and screen blood bank sample.
- Administer nonparticulate antacid <30 minutes before induction.
- May consider metoclopramide 10 mg and/or ranitidine 30 mg IV if >30 minutes prior to induction.
- In patients with high body mass index may consider the placement of a ramp to optimize patient positioning for intubation.

- If the patient is greater than 20 weeks of gestation (uterus at or above the umbilicus), it is vital to place the patient in left uterine displacement prior to induction.
- Administer indicated antibiotics.
- Perform preoxygenation with either 100% O_2 for 3 minutes or 4 to 8 vital capacity breaths.[1]
- Ensure the patient is prepped and draped, perform time-out, and confirm surgeon is ready for incision. This is done to shorten the time from induction to delivery, which minimizes the anesthetic effect on the neonate.

INDUCTION

- Initiate rapid sequence induction.
- Propofol 2.0 to 2.5 mg/kg of ideal body weight (IBW) and succinylcholine 1.0 to 1.5 mg/kg of total body weight. Etomidate 0.3 mg/kg may be used with hypovolemia.
  - Avoid opioids and benzodiazepines before delivery, as they cross the placenta and may cause neonatal respiratory depression.
- Wait ~30 to 45 seconds, then perform tracheal intubation.
  - Ideally, a senior anesthesiologist or an attending should be the intubator.
  - Airway edema associated with pregnancy, labor and preeclampsia may necessitate video laryngoscopy; this should be ready if not the first choice.
  - Endotracheal tube size 6.5 or 6.0 mm should be considered in light of airway edema.[2]
- Confirm placement and inform obstetricians that it is safe to initiate surgery.

INTRAOPERATIVE PRIOR TO DELIVERY

- Use volatile anesthetic (sevoflurane, isoflurane, or desflurane) at approximately 1 minimum alveolar concentration (MAC).
- Recommended initial ventilator settings of 6 to 8 mL/kg of IBW and a respiratory rate of 14 to 18/min.
- There is a compensatory *respiratory alkalosis* in pregnancy with a normal $PaCO_2$ of 30 mm Hg. Ventilator settings should be titrated to maintain patients near this baseline.
- Treat hypotension as necessary.

INTRAOPERATIVE AFTER DELIVERY

- Remove the wedge.
- Initiate continuous infusion of oxytocin.
  - Monitor uterine tone closely and consider boluses of Oxytocin 3 IU. If the tone is insufficient, consider early use of secondary uterotonics and consider total intravenous anesthesia instead of a volatile agent.
- Adjust maintenance anesthetic:
  - Reduce volatile anesthetic to 0.5 MAC.
  - Add 50% of nitrous oxide.
  - Consider the addition of midazolam. Pregnant women have an increased risk of intraoperative awareness.
  - Provide opioids for intraoperative and postoperative analgesia:
    - Fentanyl 100 to 200 µg.
    - Hydromorphone 0.5 to 1.0 mg.

- ○ Place temperature probe and upper body forced-air warmer.
- ○ Administer intravenous ketorolac and opioids for postoperative pain and ondansetron for nausea and vomiting.
- Pay careful attention to extubation with the patient maintaining appropriate respiratory physiology, fully awake and following commands.
  - ○ The majority of respiratory-related deaths occurred during emergence, extubation, and recovery.[3]
  - ○ Consider the placement of an oral gastric tube to empty the gastric contents if the patient did not meet NPO (nothing by mouth) guidelines or there is a concern for a full stomach.

POSTOPERATIVE

- Evaluate postoperative issues in postanesthesia care unit.
- Consider quadratus lumborum or transversus abdominis plane block for postoperative pain.

References

1. Gambee AM, Hertzka RE, Fisher DM. Preoxygenation techniques: comparison of three minutes and four breaths. *Anesth Analg.* 1987;66(5):468-470.
2. Kodali BS, Chandrasekhar S, Bulich LN, et al. Airway changes during labor and delivery. *Anesthesiology.* 2008;108(3):357-362.
3. Mhyre JM. A series of anesthesia-related maternal deaths in Michigan, 1985-2003. *Anesthesiology.* 2007;106(6):1096-1104.

49

Conversion of Labor Epidural for Cesarean Delivery

Yunping Li, MD

BACKGROUND

The incidence of intrapartum cesarean delivery (CD) varies between 8% and 20% among different hospitals. Anesthesia for intrapartum CD differs from elective CD because:

- It is often emergent or urgent.
- Usually, the patient has an existing labor epidural rather than a de novo spinal or combined spinal and epidural (CSE).
- Failure rates for conversion of labor epidural analgesia to surgical anesthesia for CD can be as high as 20%.[1]
- Postoperative CD analgesia can also be complicated for a patient who has endured both labor pain and CD pain.

Successful conversion of labor epidural analgesia to CD anesthesia is a meaningful measure of quality of care and an important clinical process to reduce the incidence of general anesthesia and ensure maternal comfort during CD.[2]

The definition of failure of conversion varies greatly in literature resulting in a great difference in the incidence of failure of conversion. Most authors define **failed conversion** as the need to perform either a repeat neuraxial procedure or general anesthesia.

THE RISKS OF FAILURE OF CONVERSION[3]

- Recurrent breakthrough pain requesting multiple epidural boluses (Odds ratio, OR 3.2)
- Urgency of CD (OR 40.4)
- Long duration of labor epidural
- Nonobstetric anesthesia specialized provider (OR 4.6)
- Second-stage arrest[4]
- Chorioamnionitis[5]

STRATEGIES FOR SUCCESSFUL CONVERSION (FIG. 49-1)

Understanding the reasons for failure will help anesthesiologists strategically plan to achieve a successful conversion. Early and active steps to prevent failure are more desirable than late recognition with the potential need for general anesthesia. The following are suggested:

- Aggressively treat breakthrough pain (Chapter 42, "Refractory Pain During Labor Epidural Analgesia").
- Replace the epidural catheter early if the sensory level does not improve with repeat boluses.
- If breakthrough pain is refractory to treatment during labor, consider replacing a new CSE in the operating room. A reduced dose of bupivacaine (0.8-1.2 mL of 0.75% hyperbaric bupivacaine) for spinal part is recommended.[6] Be aware of the risk of high spinal (Chapter 60, "High Spinal").
- A small dose of epidural dexmedetomidine (10-20 μg) may improve pain control (Chapter 6, "Dexmedetomidine").

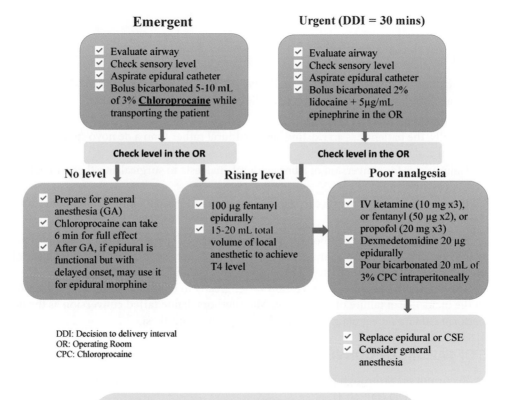

FIGURE 49-1 • Strategies for successful conversion of labor epidural for CD.

References

1. Mankowitz SK, Gonzalez FA, Smiley R. Failure to extend epidural labor analgesia for cesarean delivery anesthesia. *Anesth Analg*. 2016;123:1174-1180.

2. Desai N, Carvalho B. Conversion of labour epidural analgesia to surgical anaesthesia for emergency intrapartum caesarean section. *BJA Education*. 2020;20(1):26-31.

3. Bauer ME, Kountanis JA, Tsen LC, et al. Risk factors for failed conversion of labor epidural analgesia to cesarean delivery anesthesia: a systematic review and meta-analysis of observational trials. *Int J Obstet Anesth*. 2012;21:294-309.

4. Xu S, Sorabella L, Li Y, et al. Prolonged second stage labor: a risk factor for failed conversion from neuraxial analgesia to cesarean anesthesia. Society for Obstetric Anesthesia and Perinatology Annual Meeting 2018.

5. Katakura Y, Nagamine Y, Goto T, et al. Association of chorioamnionitis with failed conversion of epidural labor analgesia to cesarean delivery anesthesia: a retrospective cohort study. *PLoS One*. 2021;16(5):e0250596.

6. Visser WA, Dijkstra A, Albayrak M, et al. Spinal anesthesia for intrapartum cesarean delivery following epidural labor analgesia: a retrospective cohort study. *Can J Anesth*. 2009;56:577-583.

50

Hypotension After Spinal Anesthesia

Amnon A. Berger, MD, PhD

BACKGROUND

As discussed in other chapters, neuraxial anesthesia is the most common and preferred anesthetic for cesarean delivery. Induction of spinal anesthesia causes a sympathectomy leading to vasodilation and, rarely bradycardia, resulting in maternal hypotension.[1] Avoiding hypotension in parturients is important as the human placenta has minimal autoregulation, and fetal perfusion is determined solely by maternal perfusion pressure. Although serious adverse events resulting from hypotension are uncommon, hypotension following spinal anesthesia induction is associated with maternal nausea and vomiting, with fetal heart rate (HR) changes, and prolonged hypotension can lead to fetal acidosis.[2]

Coloading with crystalloids and use of vasoconstrictive agents have been shown to lower the incidence of hypotension following administration of spinal anesthesia.[3] Phenylephrine and ephedrine are most commonly used to prevent and treat spinal hypotension, largely because they are best supported by existing evidence.[2,4,5] Phenylephrine is the preferred prophylactic agent, as ephedrine crosses the placental barrier more than phenylephrine and is associated with a mild fetal acidemia of unknown significance.[2,6] The Society for Obstetric Anesthesia and Perinatology Enhanced Recovery After Cesarean Delivery guidelines recommend prophylactic phenylephrine infusion to prevent hypotension. Studies have shown that a low-dose infusion of phenylephrine reduces the incidence of hypotension and nausea after spinal from 40% to less than 10%. Small doses of ephedrine can be used to treat hypotension in women with lower HR, and bradycardia can be treated with anticholinergic drugs.[2] Emerging evidence suggest that norepinephrine, with its mild β-adrenergic activity, maintains cardiac output and may be potentially more effective in preventing hypotension without bradycardia.[4,7,8]

GOALS

- To reduce the incidence and severity of hypotension following induction of spinal anesthesia.
- To maintain maternal systolic blood pressure (SBP) $\geq$90% of a known baseline, or >100 mm Hg if a baseline is unknown.
- To improve recovery and prevent adverse maternal and neonatal effects of hypotension, such as intraoperative nausea and vomiting and fetal acidosis.

CLINICAL PRACTICE

- Intravenous (IV) fluid bolus of 10 to 15 mL/kg may be administered as a coload during spinal anesthesia, as discussed above, if there are no contraindications. We recommend using an in-line fluid warmer when administering a coload bolus.
- Aortocaval compression should be avoided by placing parturients in left uterine displacement position (30°) until the neonate has been delivered.
- Closely monitor blood pressure (BP). Most cases will not have continuous BP measurement, and we recommend cycling the noninvasive BP cuff frequently until BP stabilizes.
- Pharmacologic prophylaxis should be used. We recommend initiating a phenylephrine infusion at 0.5 mcg/kg/min (or 25-50 mcg/min) at the time of induction of spinal anesthesia. Frequent adjustments should be made to maintain SBP at target.
- Pharmacologic therapy could include bolus doses of ephedrine and phenylephrine based on maternal HR and BP. Ephedrine 10 mg is preferred if HR <70 bpm and may also provide longer-lasting effects. Phenylephrine 100 to 200 mcg can be used as a starting dose for patients with HR >90.
- Physical compression devices, such as compression bandages and pneumatic boots, can also be used, though data and efficacy are limited.

METHOD OF ADMINISTRATION

Given the nature of obstetric anesthesia, phenylephrine and ephedrine should always be available for immediate use. Prophylactic infusion should be started as soon as spinal anesthesia is induced, along with a rapid infusion of a crystalloid coload. Automatic infusion pumps should be used, and weight-based dosing is preferred.

EXCEPTIONS

A prophylactic infusion is not routinely started in parturients with hypertensive disorders of pregnancy, as this group of patients may have altered endothelial responsiveness to vasoactive agents. However, vigilance must be maintained, and SBP in patients with hypertensive disorders and pre-eclampsia should be maintained within 20% of recent blood pressures.

For labor analgesia, the lower dose of spinal local anesthetic given as part of a combined spinal epidural technique rarely causes significant hypotension. It does not require routine administration of vasopressors. However, vasopressors should be immediately available to correct hypotension if it does occur.

CONTRAINDICATIONS

- No absolute contraindications exist to the treatment of hypotension with either IV fluids or vasopressors.

References

1. Langesæter E, Dyer RA. Maternal haemodynamic changes during spinal anaesthesia for caesarean section. *Curr Opin Anaesthesiol.* 2011;3:242-248. doi:10.1097/ACO.0b013e32834588c5.
2. Kinsella SM, Carvalho B, Dyer RA, et al. International consensus statement on the management of hypotension with vasopressors during caesarean section under spinal anaesthesia. *Anaesthesia.* 2018;1:71-92.
3. Ngan Kee WD, Khaw KS, Ng FF. Prevention of hypotension during spinal anesthesia for cesarean delivery: an effective technique using combination phenylephrine infusion and crystalloid cohydration. *Anesthesiology.* 2005;4:744-750.

4. Fitzgerald JP, Fedoruk KA, Jadin SM, Carvalho B, Halpern SH. Prevention of hypotension after spinal anaesthesia for caesarean section: a systematic review and network meta-analysis of randomised controlled trials. *Anaesthesia.* 2020;1:109-121.

5. Bollag L, Lim G, Sultan P, et al. Society for Obstetric Anesthesia and Perinatology: consensus statement and recommendations for enhanced recovery after cesarean. *Anesth Analg.* 2021;5:1362-1377.

6. Ngan Kee WD, Khaw KS, Tan PE, Ng FF, Karmakar MK. Placental transfer and fetal metabolic effects of phenylephrine and ephedrine during spinal anesthesia for cesarean delivery. *Anesthesiology.* 2009;3:506-512.

7. Singh PM, Singh NP, Reschke M, et al. Vasopressor drugs for the prevention and treatment of hypotension during neuraxial anaesthesia for Caesarean delivery: a Bayesian network meta-analysis of fetal and maternal outcomes. *Br J Anaesth.* 2020;3:e95-e107.

8. Mohta M, Bambode N, Chilkoti GT, et al. Neonatal outcomes following phenylephrine or norepinephrine for treatment of spinal anaesthesia-induced hypotension at emergency caesarean section in women with fetal compromise: a randomised controlled study. *Int J Obstet Anesth.* 2022;49:103247.

51

Enhanced Recovery After Cesarean

Lindsay K. Sween, MD, MPH
Liberty G. Reforma, MD
Philip E. Hess, MD

BACKGROUND

Enhanced recovery after surgery (ERAS) care pathways were originally developed in the 1990s to 2000s for colorectal surgery. They have since been developed for many other surgical subspecialties. ERAS protocols standardize patient care throughout the perioperative period, thus improving outcomes (e.g., postoperative pain and hospital length of stay) and patient satisfaction.[1] Enhanced recovery after cesarean delivery (ERAC) care pathways provide evidence-based recommendations for preoperative, intraoperative, and postoperative maternal care.[1-4]

GOALS

- Improve patient satisfaction and outcomes.
- Reduce postoperative pain, nausea/vomiting, time to void, and time to ambulation by minimizing opioids and maximizing alternative medications and techniques.

CLINICAL PRACTICE

Table 51-1 demonstrates a sample ERAC protocol utilized at a single tertiary care academic medical center.

TABLE 51-1 • Enhanced Recovery After Cesarean Delivery at BIDMC[5]

	Scheduled Cesarean	Unscheduled Cesarean
To Whom It Applies	Patients with scheduled cesarean delivery.	Patients with unscheduled cesarean delivery (e.g., intrapartum).
NPO Guidelines	Patients should eat their last large presurgery meal prior to midnight on the night before surgery. They may have a light, low-fat snack (e.g., crackers or one slice of dry toast) up to 6 hours prior to surgery. They may have clear liquids up until 2 hours before surgery. Patients will be instructed to drink a noncarbonated, nonparticulate 45-g carbohydrate beverage (e.g., Gatorade or apple juice) up to 2 hours prior to surgery for nondiabetic patients.	Patients should be NPO (nothing by mouth) as soon as the decision for cesarean section is made. Depending on the urgency of delivery, the anesthesia and obstetric team will discuss appropriate timing based on last intake. If patients have neuraxial anesthesia during labor, their diet should be changed to clear liquids at the time of placement.
Preoperative (Anesthesia)	Anesthesia assessment	
Intraoperative (Anesthesia)	• Antibiotics within 60 minutes of skin incision. (Cephalosporin preferred. Add azithromycin if patient in labor or membranes ruptured.) • Neuraxial anesthesia is the preferred method. • Aspiration prophylaxis with nonparticulate antacid. • Appropriate patient monitoring. • IV fluid warming and increased OR temperature to at least 68°F are recommended to prevent hypothermia in patients under neuraxial anesthesia; forced air warming can be added for patient comfort, neonatal skin to skin, or during general anesthesia. • Prophylactic IV ondansetron 4 mg at the end of surgery. • Treat shivering PRN (e.g., dexmedetomidine 10 µg, IV, may repeat up to 30 µg). • First dose of ketorolac 30 mg after fascia is closed.	
Postoperative Orders	Standard medication order sets by obstetricians and anesthesia teams	
Labor & Delivery Recovery (Anesthesia)	**Pain medications:** • IV ketorolac 30 mg every 6 hours for 24 hours, then transition to PO ibuprofen 600 mg every 6 hours and acetaminophen 1 g every 8 hours. • Oxycodone 5 mg every 4 hours PRN (as needed) for severe pain (avoid opioids in first 24 hours in most cases). • Pre-emptive or rescue supplementary regional blocks as indicated by anesthesia. **Nausea medications:** • IV ondansetron 4 mg every 6 hours, PRN. • IV haloperidol 0.5-1 mg, promethazine 6.25 mg, dexamethasone 4 mg used for refractory nausea and vomiting.	

Source: Reproduced with permission from CP-PP-22 Enhanced recovery after cesarean delivery carepath. 2020. © Beth Israel Deaconess Medical Center. Accessed April 2022.

References

1. Bollag L, Lim G, Sultan P, et al. Society for Obstetric Anesthesia and Perinatology: consensus statement and recommendations for enhanced recovery after cesarean. *Anesth Analg.* 2021;132(5):1362-1377.

2. Wilson RD, Caughey AB, Wood SL, et al. Guidelines for antenatal and preoperative care in cesarean delivery: enhanced recovery after surgery society recommendations (Part 1). *Am J Obstet Gynecol.* 2018;219(6):523.e1-523.e15; https://doi .org/10.1016/j.ajog.2018.09.015

3. Caughey AB, Wood SL, Macones GA, et al. Guidelines for antenatal and preoperative care in cesarean delivery: enhanced recovery after surgery society recommendations (Part 2). *Am J Obstet Gynecol.* 2018; 219(6):533-544; https://doi.org/10.1016/j.ajog.2018.08.006

4. Macones GA, Caughey AB, Wood SL, et al. Guidelines for antenatal and preoperative care in cesarean delivery: enhanced recovery after surgery society recommendations (Part 3). *Am J Obstet Gynecol.* 2019; 221(3):247.e1-247.e9; https://doi.org/10.1016/j.ajog.2019.04.012

5. Beth Israel Deaconess Medical Center©. CP-PP-22 Enhanced recovery after cesarean delivery carepath. 2020. Accessed in April 2022.

52

External Cephalic Version

Lior Levy, MD

BACKGROUND

Approximately 3% to 4% of term fetuses present breech. Vaginal breech delivery is associated with excess risk of neonatal near miss and perinatal morbidity and mortality, compared with vaginal cephalic delivery. External cephalic version (ECV) is the manual rotation of the fetus' head to a cephalic presentation to achieve cephalic vaginal delivery and decrease cesarean delivery (CD) rates. ECV is successful about 58% of the time (40% for nulliparous and 64% for multiparous). A successful version decreases the risk of CD by about 40% in this patient population. Table 52-1 lists factors that influence success of ECV.

TIMING OF ECV

- Timing is controversial, typically between 37 and 39 weeks in the United States.
- Better success rate at 34 to 36 weeks but does not seem to lead to lower CD rates. This is likely due to the increased risk of reversion to breech. Furthermore, if an emergency CD is necessary, the baby will be preterm.
- ECV can be done in laboring patients, yet rarely successful and is discouraged once membranes are ruptured, or cervix is in advanced dilation.

TABLE 52-1 • Factors That Influence Success of ECV	
Factors That Increase Success of ECV	**Factors That Reduce Success of ECV**
• Prior vaginal delivery • Use of neuraxial anesthesia • Unengaged presenting part • Transverse lie • Earlier gestational age • Experienced obstetrician • Use of terbutaline • Black race	• Nulliparity • Strong abdominal muscles • Descent of buttocks/feet into pelvis • Anterior or lateral placenta • Posterior position of fetal back • Decreased amniotic fluid volume • Low fetal weight • Ruptured membranes • Obesity

COMPLICATIONS OF ECV

Overall, ECV has a very low complication rate (about 1%) and is considered safe.

A systematic review involving 12,995 patients shows the following complications[1]:

- Transient (6.1%) and persistent (0.2%) fetal heart rate abnormalities
- Emergency CD (0.33%)
- Vaginal bleeding (0.3%)
- Stillbirth (0.19%)
- Placental abruption (0.08%)
- Ruptured membranes and cord prolapse (0.2%)
- Fetomaternal hemorrhage (0.9%) during a version; consider giving Rhogam to the Rh-negative patients

CONTRAINDICATIONS FOR ECV

- Need for a CD regardless of fetal presentation (i.e., placenta previa)
- Antepartum bleeding within 7 days
- Placental abruption
- Abnormal fetal heart rate tracing
- Major uterine abnormality
- Multiple gestations (except delivery of the second twin)
- Severe oligohydramnios

INFLUENCE OF NEURAXIAL ANESTHESIA ON ECV[2]

- ECV can be *painful*.
- Initial concerns were that providing anesthesia for ECV would encourage excessive force. Evidence shows *spinal anesthesia decreases the force required for a successful version.*
- Multiple studies show that the use of neuraxial significantly increases the success rate of ECV (58.4% vs. 43.1%) and lowers the rate of CD (46.0% vs. 55.3%).
- No studies have shown that anesthesia increases the incidence of complications of ECV.
- Of note, two other large systematic reviews have not found that CD rates were significantly lowered with the use of neuraxial. This is due to these studies being underpowered for this outcome.
- A meta-analysis of seven studies had concluded that an anesthetic dose of local anesthetic increased the rate of success of ECV, versus an analgesic dose, which had no effect. In contrast, Chalifoux et al.[3] later published a randomized study that found that 2.5 mg bupivacaine has the same rate of successful version and CD delivery rates as 5, 7.5, and 10 mg of bupivacaine. In addition, *the time to discharge was increased by 60 minutes* with 7.5 mg and 10 mg compared to 2.5 mg.

CLINICAL PRACTICE

Encourage the use of terbutaline 0.25 mg subcutaneously, immediately prior to ECV.

Two different groups of patients present to labor and delivery for an ECV:

Group 1: Patients around 37 weeks who will be discharged home regardless of the outcome of ECV unless an emergent CD is performed. The patient is discharged once the fetal heart rate is reassuring with a reactive nonstress test and neuraxial has worn off. In this group of patients, there is an advantage to the use of a shorter-acting anesthetic.

Group 2: Patients around 39 weeks who will stay for induction of labor if the ECV is successful or CD if the ECV fails.

ANESTHETIC MANAGEMENT

We currently recommend two techniques:

- **Combined spinal and epidural** (CSE) with a full or reduced dose of 7.5 to 11.25 mg bupivacaine $\pm$ 15 to 25 µg fentanyl, no intrathecal morphine.
  - It is essential to omit neuraxial morphine in cases where the patient does not undergo CD. If the patient does not have a CD, they need to be kept in the hospital 24 hours after administration of neuraxial morphine for respiratory monitoring.
- **Epidural or dural puncture epidural** with 3% chloroprocaine.
  Be prepared for hypotension, especially if a full anesthetic dose is given.
- Left uterine displacement, hydration, and phenylephrine infusion and/or boluses.
  Be prepared for the possibility of an emergent CD for which you will need:
- Antibiotics.
- Adequate anesthesia to potentially increase the sensory level and prolong spinal anesthetic. Given the potentially emergent nature, either 2% lidocaine or 3% chloroprocaine epidurally is recommended.
- Oxytocin post-delivery.
- 3 mg Morphine epidurally.

The epidural catheter will be left in place for labor analgesia in Group 2 patients if the ECV is successful. A test dose should be given before the initiation of the labor epidural.

References

1. Grootscholten K, Kok M, Oei SG, et al. External cephalic version-related risks: a meta-analysis. *Obstet Gynecol.* 2008;112:1143-1115.
2. Magro-Malosso ER, Saccone G, Di Tommaso M, et al. Neuraxial analgesia to increase the success rate of external cephalic version: a systematic review and meta-analysis of randomized controlled trials. [Published correction appears in Am J Obstet Gynecol. 2017 Mar;216(3):315]. *Am J Obstet Gynecol.* 2016;215(3):276-286.
3. Chalifoux LA, Bauchat JR, Higgins N, et al. Effect of intrathecal bupivacaine dose on the success of external cephalic version for breech presentation: a prospective, randomized, blinded clinical trial. *Anesthesiology.* 2017;127: 625-632.

PART VIII

POST CESAREAN CARE

53

Postanesthetic Care

Yunping Li, MD
Philip E. Hess, MD

American Society of Anesthesiology (ASA) Task Force published the practice guideline for postanesthetic care in 2002.[1] The purpose of these guidelines is to improve postanesthetic care outcomes for patients who have just had anesthesia and analgesia care.

General medical supervision and coordination of patient care in the postanesthetic care unit (PACU) should be the responsibility of anesthesiologists (ASA Standard IV).[2] The communication guidelines have been developed to improve coordinated patient care during response to urgencies/emergencies in the PACU in Labor and Delivery Unit at Beth Israel Deaconess Medical Center (BIDMC). These guidelines are modified to meet the needs of the specific patient population, obstetric patients, and to exceed the ASA Standards IV for postanesthesia care.

The goals for the BIDMC guidelines are specific to:

- Encourage high-quality patient care in the PACU.
- Promote multiple teams' collaboration.
- Ensure effective communication between healthcare professionals.
- Share information and share appropriate responsibility.

BIDMC PACU care pathways include:

- The PACU Nursing Notification Pathways (Fig. 53-1)[3]
- PACU Handoff (Fig. 53-2)[4]
- PACU Postanesthesia Note (Fig. 53-3)

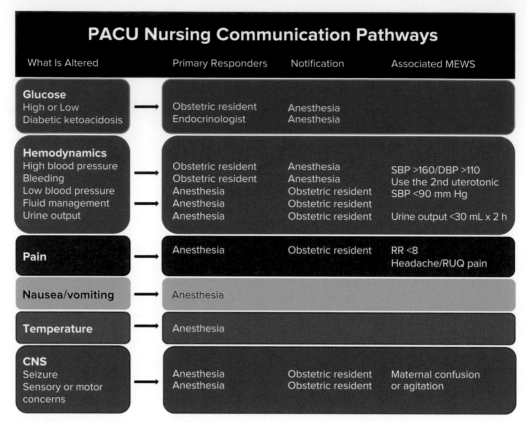

FIGURE 53-1 • PACU nursing communication pathways.

Source: Reproduced with permission from CP-OB 45 PACU Nursing Notification, 2007. © Beth Israel Deaconess Medical Center. Accessed April 2022.

CNS, central nerve system; DBP, diastolic blood pressure; MEWS, maternal early warning system; RR, respiratory rate; RUQ, right upper quadrant; SBP, systolic blood pressure.

Anesthesiologist_____ → RN _____   *(patient label)*

TYPE OF ANESTHESIA: □ Spinal   □ CSE   □ Epidural   □ Monitored Anesthesia Care
□ General   □ Intrathecal / Epidural morphine   □ TAP/QL Block

MEDICATIONS GIVEN IN OPERATING ROOMS

MEDICATION	ROUTE	DOSE	TIME	MEDICATION	ROUTE	DOSE	TIME
AMPICILLIN	IV			ACETAMINOPHEN	IV		
AZITHROMYCIN	IV			DEXMEDETOMIDINE	IV/EPIDURAL		
CEFAZOLIN	IV			FENTANYL	IV		
CLINDAMYCIN	IV			HYDROMORPHONE	IV		
GENTAMYCIN	IV			KETAMINE	IV		
				KETOROLAC	IV		
CALCIUM	IV			MIDAZOLAM	IV		
CARBOPROST	IM						
MISOPROSTOL	PR			DEXAMETHASONE	IV		
OXYTOCIN BOLUS	IV			HALOPERIDOL	IV		
METHYLERGONOVINE	IM			PROMETHAZINE	IV		
TRANEXAMIC ACID	IV			ONDANSETRON	IV		

INPUTS	TOTAL
LACTATE/NORMAL SALINE	
5% ALBUMIN	
RED BLOOD CELL	
PLATELET	
CRYOPRECIPITATE	
CELL SAVER	
PLASMALYTE	

OUTPUTS	TOTAL
QUANTITATIVE BLOOD LOSS	
ESTIMATED BLOOD LOSS	
URINE	
EMESIS	
ORAL-GASTRIC TUBE OUTPUT	

Significant intraoperative events?

Postoperative concerns?   □ Check labs?   □ Pain?   □ Hypotension?
□ Hypothermia?   □ Nausea & vomiting?
□ Epidural left in place   □ Return the blood cooler if the patient is stable
□ Other

FIGURE 53-2 • BIDMC PACU handoff.
Source: Reproduced with permission from CP-OB 57 PACU Nursing Handoff, 2021. © Beth Israel Deaconess Medical Center. Accessed April 2022.

BIDMC POSTANESTHESIA NOTE

POSTOPERATION OPTIONS

○ Not eligible for postoperative assessment
○ Intensive Care Unit
○ Postanesthesia Care Unit

Vital Signs Appropriate
□ Yes   □ No

Respiratory Function Appropriate; Airway patent
□ Yes   □ No

Cardiovascular Function and Hydration Status Appropriate
□ Yes   □ No

Pain Control Satisfactory
□ Yes   □ No

Nausea and Vomiting Control Satisfactory
□ Yes   □ No

Patient Alertness
□ Patient awake and alert and participates in evaluation
□ Patient sleepy, but easily arousable and responsive and participated in evaluation

NEURAXIAL BLOCK

□ No   □ Yes Modified Bromage Score
          Description
          1- Complete block (unable to move feet or knees)
          2- Almost complete block (able to move feet only)
          3- Partial block (just able to move knees)
          4- Detectable weakness in hip flexion (between scores 3 and 5)
          5- No detectable weakness of hip flexion while supine (full flexion of knees)
          6- Able to perform partial knee bend

COMPLICATIONS

□ No complications   □ Complications occurred

COMMENTS

FIGURE 53-3 • BIDMC postanesthesia note.
Source: Reproduced with permission from Talis. PACU Post Anesthesia Note. © Beth Israel Deaconess Medical Center. Accessed April 2022.

References

1. American Society of Anesthesiologists. Practice guidelines for postanesthetic care. A report by the American Society of Anesthesiology Task Force on Postanesthetic Care. *Anesthesiology*. 2002;96:742-752.

2. American Society of Anesthesiologists. Standards for postanesthesia care. Last amended October 23, 2019. https://www.asahq.org/standards-and-guidelines/standards-for-postanesthesia-care.

3. Beth Israel Deaconess Medical Center PPGD©. CP-OB 45 PACU Nursing Notification, 2007. Accessed April 2022.

4. Beth Israel Deaconess Medical Center PPGD©. CP-OB 57 PACU Nursing Handoff, 2021. Accessed April 2022.

54

Neuraxial Morphine

Merry I. Colella, MD

BACKGROUND

- Neuraxial morphine (intrathecal or epidural) has been used since the early 1980s to provide safe and effective postpartum postsurgical pain relief.[1,2]
- Respiratory depression associated with neuraxial morphine is extremely rare. It occurs with an average time of onset of 8 to 12 hours after neuraxial morphine installation.[1]
  - Vigilant monitoring of the patient's respiratory status for 24 hours after injection.
  - Respiratory depression is most often associated with the use of supplemental narcotics or sedatives.
- For breastfeeding patients, the newborn is not appreciably affected by morphine excretion in the colostrum after neuraxial administration of morphine.
- Only administer neuraxial morphine when the postpartum floor has the capability to monitor the patients and monitoring policy is in place.

PROCEDURE FOR IMPLEMENTATION

- It is prohibited to administer any opioids or sedatives for the first 24 hours after neuraxial morphine installation. Please discuss with the obstetric anesthesiologist if the patient needs an early dose of opioid.
- Document the dose, time, and route of neuraxial morphine using the obstetric anesthesia neuraxial morphine order set.
- This order set should also include orders for:
  - The protocol of monitoring respiratory status.
  - Ketorolac and acetaminophen for the first 24 hours postsurgery for prevention of breakthrough pain.
  - Naloxone (both single dose and infusion as needed) for management of severe pruritus, respiratory depression, or oversedation.
  - Antiemetics for management of nausea and vomiting.
- Inform the recovery room nurse when giving the report that the patient has received neuraxial morphine.
- Hand over the neuraxial morphine monitoring form to the recovery room nurse and be sure to fill out:
  - Date, time, and route of morphine administration.
  - Date, time, and mode of delivery.

POSTPARTUM CARE AND MONITORING

- The monitoring modality and frequency depends on the dose of neuraxial morphine (Table 54-1). The patients at high risk for respiratory depression require higher level of monitoring.[3] The patients include:
  - Patients who received any additional opioid for breakthrough pain.
  - Morbidly obese patients.
  - Patients diagnosed with obstructive sleep apnea.
  - Patients who have received or are still receiving an infusion of magnesium sulfate for treatment of preeclampsia.
- The obstetric anesthesiology team should be consulted within the first 24 hours of morphine administration to manage breakthrough pain or adverse effects of neuraxial morphine.
- Please discuss with the attending anesthesiologist regarding the treatment plan for breakthrough pain.

MANAGEMENT OF BREAKTHROUGH PAIN

- Orders should be entered at the time of morphine administration for ketorolac and acetaminophen **round-the-clock dosing** for the first 24 hours postsurgery.
- Patients undergoing cesarean after labor are at high risk for persistent pain despite use of neuraxial morphine. Consider a transversus abdominis plane (TAP) or quadratus lumborum (QL) block prior to transfer of patient to the postpartum unit.[4]
- If the patient declines a TAP/QL block, or has breakthrough pain despite peripheral nerve block, ketorolac and acetaminophen, administration of an additional narcotic may be considered.
  - If the patient is on the postpartum floor, give a **single dose of oxycodone** (5-10 mg), and ensure that the patient is monitored for appropriate respiration using telemetry/pulse oximetry.
  - If the patient is in the recovery room, consider using small dose of intravenous fentanyl or morphine while continuing to monitor.
- Initiate patient-controlled intravenous opioids when neuraxial dosing appears to not have been delivered.

TABLE 54-1 • Society for Obstetric Anesthesia and Perinatology Respiratory Monitoring Recommendations[3]	
Neuraxial Morphine Dose	**Respiratory Monitoring**
Ultra-low dose: IT ≤50 µg or epidural ≤**1 mg**	None
Low dose: IT 50-150 µg or epidural 1-3 mg	Monitor respiratory rate and sedation score q2h for 12 hours
High dose: IT >150 µg or epidural >3 mg or patients with risk factors	Monitor respiratory rate, sedation score +/− pulse oximetry q1h for 12 hours then q2h for another 12 hours

IT, intrathecal.

Source: Bauchat JR, Weiniger CF, Sultan P, et al. Society for Obstetric Anesthesia and Perinatology consensus statement: monitoring recommendations for prevention and detection of respiratory depression associated with administration if neuraxial morphine for cesarean delivery analgesia. Anesthe Analg. 2019;129:458-474.

MANAGEMENT OF OTHER ISSUES

- **Moderate to severe pruritus:**
  - Exclude other possible causes of itching.
  - Orders should be entered at the time of morphine administration for:
    - Naloxone bolus, 40 to 80 µg IV, may be repeated after 5 minutes, if necessary, for a maximum total of 3 boluses.
    - Naloxone IV infusion, to be started if severe pruritus recurs after 3 boluses. Infuse for 2 hours at a rate of 200 µg/h.
    - Infusion should be stopped, and obstetric anesthesiology team called if pruritus persists, or if pain returns.
- **Nausea/vomiting:**
  - Orders should be entered at the time of morphine administration for multiple antiemetics, including ondansetron as a first-line agent, promethazine 6.25 mg IV as a second-line agent, and haloperidol 0.5 mg IV as a third-line agent.
- **Respiratory depression or oversedation/somnolence:**
  - The obstetric anesthesiology team should be called immediately to bedside for evaluation.
  - Naloxone bolus of 40 to 80 µg IV from the obstetric anesthesia order set should be administered by the bedside nurse immediately.

References

1. Crowgey TR, Dominguez JE, Peterson-Layne C, et al. A retrospective assessment of the incidence of respiratory depression after neuraxial morphine administration for postcesarean delivery analgesia. *Anesth Analg.* 2013;117:1368-1370.
2. Practice Guidelines for the prevention, detection, and management of respiratory depression associated with neuraxial opioid administration. An updated report by the American Society of Anesthesiologists Task Force on Neuraxial Opioids and the American Society of Regional Anesthesia and Pain Medicine. *Anesthesiology.* 2016;124(3):535-552.
3. Bauchat JR, Weiniger CF, Sultan P, et al. Society for Obstetric Anesthesia and Perinatology consensus statement: monitoring recommendations for prevention and detection of respiratory depression associated with administration if neuraxial morphine for cesarean delivery analgesia. *Anesthe Analg.* 2019;129:458-474.
4. Li Y, Ballard H, Carani JL, et al. Transversus abdominis plane block in parturients undergoing intrapartum cesarean delivery. *J Anesth Perioper Med.* 2019;6:15-22.

55

Analgesia After Cesarean Delivery

Minxian Liang, MD
Justin K. Stiles, MD

BACKGROUND

Cesarean delivery (CD) is the most common surgical procedure in the world.[1] Inadequate pain control can interfere with care for the neonate, negatively affects bonding and breastfeeding between mother and newborn, and is an unsatisfactory anesthetic outcome.[2,3] Multimodal analgesia is an ideal approach.

GOALS

- Early ambulation
- Unhindered care for newborn
- Minimal side effects: nausea, sedation, pruritus
- Safe with breastfeeding

CLINICAL PRACTICE

Multimodal analgesia can include (Table 55-1):
- Opioid: neuraxial versus systemic
- Nonsteroidal anti-inflammatory drugs (NSAIDs)
- Acetaminophen
- Ketamine
- Dexmedetomidine
- Peripheral nerve block: quadratus lumborum (QL) or transverse abdominis plane (TAP) block
- Oral gabapentin
- Low thoracic epidural

METHOD OF ADMINISTRATION

- Opioid
  - Neuraxial opioids: the most effective form of postoperative analgesia for CD.[3] It is superior to systemic opioids after CD.
    - Preservative-free morphine: last up to 24 hours.
    - Dose: Intrathecal: 150 to 250 µg; epidural: 3 mg after cord clamp.

- Systemic opioids: hydromorphone patient control analgesia (PCA) preferred for patients unable to receive neuraxial morphine (e.g., general anesthesia, patients with opioid use disorders).
- NSAIDs
  - Medication choice and dose: ketorolac 15 to 30 mg IV Q6H for 24 hours then ibuprofen 600 mg PO (by mouth) Q6H. Round-the-clock order preferred over prn.
- Acetaminophen
  - Acetaminophen 1 g PO or IV in the recovery room.
  - Then 1 g PO Q8H. Round-the-clock order preferred over prn.
- Ketamine
  - 20 to 40 mg IV as a supplement for general anesthesia.
  - For chronic opioid use patient, may require ketamine infusion, dose 0.2 to 0.3 mg/kg/h post-operatively (consult acute pain service).
- Dexmedetomidine
  - For chronic opioid use patients, consider avoiding intrathecal morphine and replacing with 10 μg intrathecal dexmedetomidine.
  - For intrapartum CD, may consider administer 10 to 20 μg dexmedetomidine via epidural in the patients who experienced multiple breakthrough pain during labor.
- QL/TAP block
  - Ultrasound guided peripheral nerve blocks: 0.25% bupivacaine 15 to 20 mL on each side (limit 0.25 mg/kg bupivacaine). It covers T6-L1 nerve roots involved in lower abdominal surgeries, possibly 12 to 16 hours coverage.
  - Cautious use after cesarean under epidural anesthesia (local anesthetic toxicity).
- Gabapentin PO
  - Single dose of 300 mg PO preoperatively.[4]

TABLE 55-1 • Analgesia Options for Post-CD				
Medication	Elective CD	Intrapartum CD	CD Under General Anesthesia	CD in Opioid Use Disorder Patients
Acetaminophen	✓	✓	✓	✓
Ketorolac/NSAIDs	✓	✓	✓	✓
Neuraxial morphine	✓	✓		
QL/TAP block		±	✓	✓
PCA			✓	✓
Dexmedetomidine		±		✓
Gabapentin			±	✓
Ketamine			±	±
Low thoracic epidural				±

CD, cesarean delivery; NSAIDs, nonsteroidal anti-inflammatory drugs; PCA, patient control analgesia.

References

1. Visser GHA, Ayres-de-Campos D, Barnea ER, et al. FIGO position paper: how to stop the caesarean section epidemic. *Lancet.* 2018;392(10155):1286-1287.

2. Carvalho B, Cohen SE, Lipman SS, et al. Patient preferences for anesthesia outcomes associated with cesarean delivery. *Anesth Analg.* 2005;101:1182.

3. Bauchat JR, Weiniger CF, Sultan P, et al. Society for Obstetric Anesthesia and Perinatology consensus statement: monitoring recommendations for prevention and detect of respiratory depression associated with administration of neuraxial morphine for cesarean delivery analgesia. *Anesth Analg.* 2019;129:458-474.

4. Moore A, Costello J, Wieczorek P, Shah V, Taddio A, Carvalho JC. Gabapentin improves postcesarean delivery pain management: a randomized, placebo-controlled trial. *Anesth Analg.* 2011;112(1):167-173.

56

Breastfeeding After Anesthesia

Joan E. Spiegel, MD

BACKGROUND

Breastfeeding is recommended by the World Health Organization as the best source of nutrition for infants, with potential health benefits for both mother and child. Anesthesiologists are frequently asked about the safety of medications in breastfeeding infants and time from anesthesia and surgery to resuming breastfeeding.

Transfer of medications from the maternal system to breastmilk depends upon protein binding, lipid solubility, molecular weight, pKa, and maternal plasma levels of the drug. Medications that are highly lipid soluble, less protein bound, low molecular weight, and a higher pKa will have a higher rate of transfer to breastmilk. Passage is largely via passive diffusion as very few drugs are actively transported into breastmilk.

Most medications can cross into colostrum (immediately after delivery) because the intracellular junctions between lactocytes close by 48 to 72 hours postpartum. However, because colostrum volume is low and neonate intake is also low, risk of potentially "harmful" breastmilk to the infant starts after day 3 of life.

The RID (%) (Relative Infant Dose)

$$\text{RID} = \frac{\text{estimated daily infant dose via breastmilk (mg/kg/day)}}{\text{infant therapeutic dose (mg/kg/day)}} \times 100$$

RID levels less than 10% are generally considered safe. Fortunately, almost all anesthetics and drugs used in delivering a multimodal anesthetic have RIDs significantly less than 10%. A few drugs not recommended for breastfeeding mothers include **codeine, tramadol, amphetamines, chemotherapy agents, ergotamine, and statins**.

Narcotics are the most concerning, but improved pain translates to better breastfeeding outcomes in the postpartum period. Narcotics used for procedural anesthesia and post-surgical pain relief in breastfeeding mothers can be administered safely within reason. There are very few rigorous studies regarding procedural sedation and anesthesia in breastfeeding mothers, and information guiding recommendations is gathered from small sample observations, case studies, and animal studies which may not translate to humans; thus guidelines are based upon expert opinion or GRADE III and IV quality of evidence (poor).

CLINICAL PRACTICE AND GUIDELINES FOR ANESTHESIOLOGISTS[1-5]

Multimodal pain regiment is a pharmacologic method which combines various medications at their lowest appropriate doses for effective pain relief, including local anesthetics, opioids, acetaminophen, nonsteroidal anti-inflammatory drugs (NSAIDs), and alpha-2 agonists.

- Drugs with high protein binding, low RID, and shorter half-life are preferred.
- Commonly available medications in the perioperative period (midazolam, fentanyl, propofol, inhalational anesthetics, and antiemetics) are considered safe, especially when single doses are used, and when an infant is healthy and term.
- Resume breastfeeding when the breastfeeding mother is awake and alert following anesthesia. (Resumption of maternal mentation is an indication that medications have redistributed from the plasma and entered adipose where they are more slowly released.)
- If there is concern by the caregiver and/or breastfeeding mother about transfer of medications to breastmilk, the mother can be advised to store breastmilk in the freezer until the infant is older or dilute the breastmilk with "unadulterated" breastmilk or formula to reduce transmission of medications to the infant.
  - This is especially important if the infant or newborn is at risk for apnea.
- Women do not need to be advised to discard breastmilk following procedures or delivery unless they were administered medications that are not recommended, or that clearly exceeded the recommended dosages, and/or the infant is at high risk for apnea (as in prematurity).
- Following general anesthesia, a breastfeeding mother should be monitored by a responsible adult and avoid co-sleeping with her infant for a 24-hour period.
- These guidelines are for mothers that are not opioid dependent. In such patients, advice and recommendations would be on a case-by-case basis. Although breastfeeding would not be contraindicated, these infants will have narcotic withdrawal and consultation with a pediatrician would be recommended (Chapter 16, "Opioid Use Disorders").

MEDICATIONS AND BREASTFEEDING (TABLE 56-1)

TABLE 56-1 • Common Anesthetic Medications and Safety in Breastfeeding		
Medications	**Routes of Administration**	**Safety Considerations**
Acetaminophen	Oral, rectal, IV	Transfer to milk is relatively low; RID 6-24%
Meperidine	IV	Should be avoided
Fentanyl and remifentanil	IV	Ideal as transfer is low and oral bioavailability is low; RID 1%
Hydromorphone and hydrocodone	IV	RID 3%; long half-life warrants judicious use
Morphine	IV, PCA	Reasonable option when narcotics required; passage to milk and oral bioavailability are low but RID is 9% and caution is recommended
Nalbuphine and butorphanol	IV/IM	Inactive metabolites, low infant RID, low oral bioavailability make these very reasonable choices
Hydrocodone	PO	Safe but should limit the daily maternal dose to 30 mg
Oxycodone	PO	Commonly used post-cesarean delivery; limit daily dose to 30 mg

TABLE 56-1 • Common Anesthetic Medications and Safety in Breastfeeding		
Medications	**Routes of Administration**	**Safety Considerations**
Codeine	PO	**Not** recommended for breastfeeding mothers due to excessive infant sedation (as a prodrug, metabolism via CYP2D6 makes its effects unpredictable in mother and infant)
Methadone	PO	Although breastfeeding is encouraged in women with chronic opioid dependence, each case must be considered separately
Tramadol	PO	**Not** recommended for use in the United States
NSAIDs	Oral, IV, rectal	Ibuprofen has a very short half-life with little milk transfer; aspirin at 81 mg is safe; PO ketorolac is very safe; IV ketorolac not recommended by manufacturer >72 hours postpartum Should be avoided in mother's infants with ductal-dependent cardiac lesions All oral NSAIDs considered safe at standard doses for use less than 1 week
Ketamine	IV	No supporting studies; unknown RID; can use small doses
Propofol and thiopental	IV	Very safe; RID 0.1%
Inhaled anesthetics (sevoflurane, isoflurane, nitrous oxide)	Inhalational	Short half-lives; safe to resume breastfeeding after administration
Midazolam	IV	RID 0.3%; safe in routine doses
Neuromuscular blocking agents (succinylcholine, rocuronium)	IV	Safe as they have low lipid solubility and distributed in the extracellular fluid volume
Sugammadex and neostigmine	IV	RID 0.1% for neostigmine; unknown for sugammadex; considered safe
Dexmedetomidine	IV, IV infusion	Safe; when used as an adjunct during cesarean delivery, the RID 0.04-0.09%
Clonidine	Epidural infusion or single dose	Single epidural dose considered safe; no studies on infusion and breastfeeding
Vasopressors (ephedrine, phenylephrine)	IV, IM	Poor oral bioavailability; safe when used intraoperatively for BP management
Local anesthetics	Epidural, regional, local	These large, polarized molecules have low oral bioavailability and are poorly transferred to breastmilk; RID 0.1%
Gabapentin	PO	Useful for multimodal pain management; gabapentin preferred over pregabalin due to less transfer to breastmilk; RID 3%
Pregabalin	PO	See gabapentin
Antiemetics	IV, PO	Ondansetron, dexamethasone, metoclopramide preferred as they are less sedating Prochlorperazine, promethazine, and scopolamine may result in sedation if used repeatedly

BP, blood pressure; IM, intramuscular; IV, intravenous; NSAIDs, nonsteroidal anti-inflammatory drugs; PCA, patient-controlled analgesia; PO, by mouth; RID, relative infant dose.

References

1. Martin E, Vickers B, Landau R, Reece-Stremtan S. ABM Clinical Protocol #28, Peripartum Analgesia and Anesthesia for the Breastfeeding Mother. *Breastfeed Med.* 2018;13(3):164-171.

2. Reece-Stremtan S, Campos M, Kokajko L; Academy of Breastfeeding Medicine. ABM Clinical Protocol #15: Analgesia and Anesthesia for the Breastfeeding Mother. *Breastfeed Med.* 2017;12(9):500-506.

3. Mitchell J, Jones E, Winkley S, Kinsella M. Guideline on anaesthesia and sedation in breastfeeding women 2020. *Anaesthesia.* 2020;75(11):1482-1493.

4. ASA Statement on Resuming Breastfeeding after Anesthesia. Committee of Origin: Obstetric Anesthesia. Approved by the House of Delegates on October 23, 2019. https://www.asahq.org/standards-and-guidelines/statement-on-resuming-breastfeeding-after-anesthesia.

5. Cobb B, Liu R, Valentine E, Onuoha O. Breastfeeding after anesthesia: a review for anesthesia providers regarding the transfer of medications into breastmilk. *Transl Perioper Pain Med.* 2015;1(2):1-7.

57

Side Effects of Neuraxial Opioids

Galina V. Korsunsky, MD

BACKGROUND

Neuraxial morphine is the most common long-acting opioid for prolonged analgesia after a cesarean delivery.[1] However, it is associated with pruritus and postoperative nausea and vomiting (PONV).[1,2] Both of these side effects are common after neuraxial morphine, and the side effects are more common with intrathecal doses greater than 150 μg. Few parturients experience a severe form of pruritus, PONV or both, and would rather experience pain than pruritus and/or PONV; thus, it is important to treat both in a timely manner.

PRURITUS[3]

The reported incidence of pruritus is between 30% and 100%, making it the most common side effect post-cesarean delivery. The pruritus is often localized to the trunk and facial areas innervated by the trigeminal nerve. The exact mechanism is unknown. It is thought to be due to interaction between neuraxial opioids and 5-Hydroxytryptamine subtype 3 (5-HT3) receptors in the dorsal horn of the spinal cord and the spinal tract of the trigeminal nerve in the medulla. Activation of the mu- and kappa-opioid receptors in the same location is believed also to cause pruritus. Importantly, pruritus after neuraxial morphine administration is not due to histamine release.

No single agent has been found to be completely effective in preventing or treating intrathecal opioid-associated pruritus. Several classes of medications can be used to treat pruritus. In women with a history of severe intrathecal morphine-induced pruritus, other analgesic modalities should be considered.

Prophylaxis (if history of severe pruritus):
1. Consider minimal effective intrathecal morphine dose of 100 μg or morphine via epidural (3 mg) instead of intrathecal route.
2. Consider neuraxial dexmedetomidine (Chapter 6, "Dexmedetomidine").[3]
3. Avoid neuraxial morphine, and discuss use of oral/intravenous (IV) opioids.
4. Use regional techniques with bupivacaine such as transversus abdominis plane or quadratus lumborum blocks.

Treatment:
1. Assess the patient, often assurance is a good start before treatment.
2. Nalbuphine (partial mu-receptor agonist/antagonist) 2.5 mg IV. Studies have shown that doses may be repeated up to 7.5 mg total dose without an effect on analgesia.

3. Naloxone 40 to 80 μg IV or infusion of 0.25 to 2.4 μg/kg/h; be aware of reversal of analgesia.
4. Ondansetron (5-HT3 receptors antagonist) 4 to 8 mg IV.[4-8]
5. Dexmedetomidine 10 μg IV.

Diphenhydramine does NOT improve pruritus associated with neuraxial opioids but will worsen sedation.

POST-CESAREAN DELIVERY NAUSEA AND VOMITING[9]

PONV are common side effects following cesarean delivery under neuraxial anesthesia, with incidence up to 60% to 80%. Etiology is multifactorial. Nausea and vomiting associated with intrathecal opioids are due to their vascular uptake and are dose related. There are dopaminergic, muscarinic, serotonergic, histaminergic, neurokinin-1, and opioid receptors in the central nervous system, particularly in the chemoreceptor trigger zone on the floor of the fourth ventricle and the vomiting center in the lateral reticular formation. Providers should use several classes of medications targeting these receptors in preventing and treating intrathecal opioid-induced nausea and vomiting.

Prophylaxis:
1. Ondansetron 4 mg IV (5HT3).
2. Dexamethasone 4 to 8 mg IV (slow onset).
3. Avoid scopolamine patch (anticholinergic) in breastfeeding women.
4. Maintain baseline blood pressure.[10]
5. Consider decreasing the dose to a minimal effective intrathecal morphine dose of 100 μg or avoiding morphine if there is a history of intractable PONV.
6. Consider regional techniques.

Treatment:
1. Ondansetron 4 to 8 mg IV. Repeat dose within 4 to 6 hours of prophylactic ondansetron is not recommended.
2. Second-line agents:
    a. Haloperidol 0.5 to 1 mg IV.
    b. Promethazine 6.25 mg IV.
3. Low-dose propofol (20 mg IV).
4. Dexmedetomidine (slow onset).
5. Lorazepam 0.5 to 1 mg IV.

References

1. Dominguez JE, Habib AS. Prophylaxis and treatment of the side-effects of neuraxial morphine analgesia following cesarean delivery. *Curr Opin Anaesthesiol.* 2013;26(3):288-295.

2. Yurashevic M, Habib AS. Monitoring, prevention and treatment of side effects of long acting neuraxial opioids for post-cesarean analgesia. *Int J Obstet Anesth.* 2019;39:117-128.

3. Mo Y, Qiu S. Effects of dexmedetomidine in reducing post-cesarean adverse reactions. *Exp Ther Med.* 2017;14(3):2036-2039.

4. Bonnet MP, Marret E, Josserand J, Mercier FJ. Effect of prophylactic 5-HT3 receptor antagonists on pruritus induced by neuraxial opioids: a quantitative systematic review. *Br J Anaesth.* 2008;101(3):311-319.

5. Kyriakides K, Hussain SK, Hobbs GJ. Management of opioid-induced pruritus: a role for 5-HT3 antagonists? *Br J Anaesth.* 1999;82(3):439-441.

6. Ganesh A, Maxwell LG. Pathophysiology and management of opioid-induced pruritus. *Drugs.* 2007;67(16):2323-2333.

7. Kung AT, Yang X, Li Y, et al. Prevention versus treatment of intrathecal morphine-induced pruritus with ondansetron. *Int J Obstet Anesth.* 2014;23(3):222-226.

8. Koju RB, Gurung BS, Dongol Y. Prophylactic administration of ondansetron in prevention of intrathecal morphine-induced pruritus and post-operative nausea and vomiting in patients undergoing caesarean section. *BMC Anesthesiol.* 2015;15:18.

9. George RB, Allen TK, Habib AS. Serotonin receptor antagonists for the prevention and treatment of pruritus, nausea, and vomiting in women undergoing cesarean delivery with intrathecal morphine: a systematic review and meta-analysis. *Anesth Analg.* 2009;109(1):174-182.

10. George RB, McKeen DM, Dominguez JE, et al. A randomized trial of phenylephrine infusion versus bolus for nausea and vomiting during cesarean in obese women. *Can J Anaesth.* 2018;65(3):254-262.

58

Hypothermia After Neuraxial Morphine

Philip E. Hess, MD

BACKGROUND

Intrathecal morphine can produce hypothermia after cesarean delivery, likely due to a central effect on opioid receptor for thermoregulation. The incidence is about 6% to 7% in elective cesarean cases and may be dose dependent.[1] In a randomized double-blind controlled study, all parturients received spinal anesthesia containing 150 μg morphine or normal saline in addition to 10 to 12 mg bupivacaine for cesarean delivery. In both groups, a significant decrease in core temperature was noted. The patients in morphine group had lower temperature and longer duration of temperature decrease.[2] Prompt management of morphine-induced hypothermia can improve patient's comfort. After lorazepam administration, immediate cessation of symptoms and an increase to normothermia temperature within 90 minutes were often observed.[1] Untreated hypothermia may last up to 6 hours.

DIAGNOSIS

- Core temperature $<35.8°C$ ($<96.4°F$).
- **Paradoxical** symptoms: diaphoresis, subjectively feeling of being hot.
- Can be sedated or feel dizzy.
- Hypothermia is usually identified after cesarean delivery while in the recovery room.

TREATMENT[1]

- Conservative treatment: In mild cases, warm blankets, heating lamps, and Bair hugger forced hot air warmer; however, patients often feel uncomfortable with heat.
- Medication: For moderate and severe hypothermia, lorazepam 0.5 mg, intravenously, may be repeated once.
- Naloxone 40 to 80 μg can also be effective in some patients.

References

1. Hess PE, Snowman CE, Wang J. Hypothermia after cesarean delivery and its reversal with lorazepam. *Int J Obstet Anesth.* 2005;14(4):279-283.
2. Hui CK, Lin CH, Lau HP, et al. A randomised double-blind controlled study evaluating the hypothermic effect of 150 μg morphine during spinal anaesthesia for caesarean section. *Anaesthesia.* 2006;61:29-31.

PART IX
ANESTHETIC COMPLICATIONS

59

Intrathecal Catheter

Idris Mohammed, MD
Yunping Li, MD

BACKGROUND

Intrathecal (IT) catheters, also known as *continuous spinal anesthesia*, are a reliable and effective neuraxial technique.[1] Except in select cases, an intentional IT catheter is not recommended for labor analgesia due to the potential risks of high/total spinal anesthesia or devastating medication errors (Chapter 60, "High Spinal").[2] Here, the chapter focuses on the strategy and management of unintentional IT catheters in obstetric patients (Fig. 59-1).

POTENTIAL INDICATIONS FOR IT CATHETER

Consider insert an IT catheter after an unintentional dural puncture with a large bore epidural needle in the following scenarios:

- Difficult placement (multiple attempts, morbid obesity, marked scoliosis, history of back surgery potentially affecting the epidural space)
- Inability to position
- Near delivery
- Non-reassuring fetal heart rate tracing

SAFETY PRECAUTIONS FOR IT CATHETERS

To ensure safety when working with an IT catheter, please pay attention to:

- Label the IT catheter and inform the anesthesia team, the nurse, and the obstetrician.
- Use the filter for the administration of medications.
- Suggest using local anesthetic and opioid at low concentrations for IT catheter infusion.
- Check sensory and motor blockage diligently and adjust the IT infusion rate accordingly.

IDENTIFICATION OF MISPLACED EPIDURAL CATHETERS

Failure to identify an IT catheter can lead to a dangerously high spinal level or total spinal. This can lead to hypotension and poor perfusion of the fetus or emergent intubation outside the operating room and possible maternal aspiration. The importance of careful aspiration of an epidural catheter and performing a test dose cannot be overemphasized (Chapter 40, "Test Dose"). When managing an epidural catheter, consider **every bolus as a test dose**.

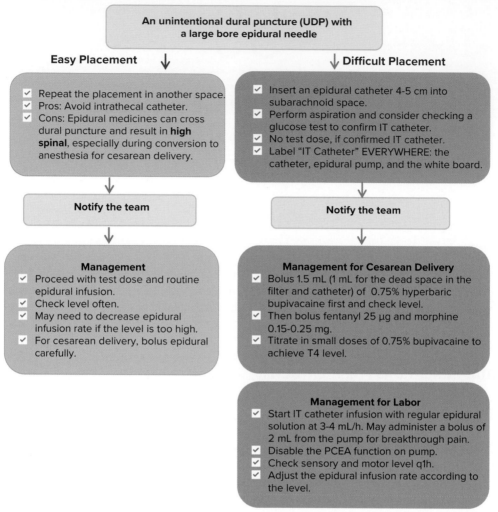

FIGURE 59-1 • Strategy and management of unintentional intrathecal catheter. IT, intrathecal; PCEA, patient-controlled epidural analgesia.

On rare occasions, an epidural catheter can be freely aspirated after prolonged infusion. The differential for this can be elicited from a glucose test and a physical exam. If the glucose test is positive, this may be explained by the catheter being placed in Tarlov cyst. If the glucose test is negative, this may represent the local accumulation of epidural solution—further aspiration attempts are typically negative. In physical exam, the patient usually lacks dense motor block in low extremities.

The differential diagnosis of IT catheter is summarized in Table 59-1.

TABLE 59-1 • Characteristics of Intrathecal, Subdural, and Epidural Catheters			
	Intrathecal	**Subdural**	**Epidural**
Aspiration of CSF	Yes	No	No
Test Dose	Dense sensory and motor block	Extensive spread (may involve the cranial nerves)	Limited spread
CSF Glucose	Positive	Negative	Negative
Onset	Fast and bilateral	Slow and variable	Slow
Hypotension	More frequent	Variable hypotension[3]	Minimal hypotension
Block Characteristics[3]	Dense sensory and motor block	Extensive sensory block Variable sympathetic and motor block (depending on dose) Unilateral or patchy block more common	Spread in a dermatomal fashion
Cranial Nerve Involvement	Only if total spinal	Frequent cranial involvement with Horner's syndrome,[4] Trigeminal nerve involved, LOC	Unlikely
Sacral Nerves	Blocked	Usually spared	Usually spared
Recovery	2-4 hours	Usually 2 hours	Early
Lubenow Criteria for Subdural Catheter[3,5] **(Two Major and One Minor)**		Major criteria Negative aspiration Extensive sensory/motor block Minor criteria Delayed onset >10 minutes Variable motor block Sympathectomy out of proportion to the dose given	

CSF, cerebrospinal fluid; LOC, loss of consciousness.

References

1. Tao W, Grant EN, Craig MG, et al. Continuous spinal analgesia for labor and delivery: an observational study with a 23-gauge spinal catheter. *Anesth Analg.* 2015;121:1290-1294.

2. Moaveni D. Management of intrathecal catheters in the obstetric patient. *BJA Education.* 2020;20(7):216-219.

3. Lubenow T, Keh-Wong E, Kristof K, et al. Inadvertent subdural injection: a complication of an epidural block. *Anesth Analg.* 1988;67:175-179.

4. Chua KJ, Cernadas M. Atypical presentation of subdural block resulting in Horner's syndrome and loss of consciousness. *BMJ case reports.* 2021;14(9):e242622.

5. Agarwal D, Mohta M, Tyagi A, et al. Subdural block and the anaesthetist. *Anaesth Intensive Care.* 2010;38:20-26.

60

High Spinal

Yunping Li, MD

INTRODUCTION

The definition of a high neuraxial block (High Spinal) is the presence of motor blockade above the intended level and which may require tracheal intubation for airway protection (Chapter 31, "Quality Indicators").[1] High neuraxial block was the leading cause of anesthesia-related maternal death,[2] and the leading cause of legal claims for maternal death or permanent brain injury filed between 1990 and 2003.[3] The incidence of high neuraxial block in obstetric anesthesia is 1:4336 in a complication repository of 257,000 anesthetics, the highest incidence in all serious anesthesia-related complications.[1]

These facts highlight the significance of avoidance, recognition, and prompt treatment of this devastating complication. High spinal or total spinal can be managed effectively to ensure patient safety if the anesthesiologist remains vigilant and responds quickly.

CAUSES OF HIGH SPINAL

- Wrong dose in wrong space: Unrecognized intrathecal catheter—immediate onset.
- Subdural catheter—delayed or immediate onset.
- Spinal after failed epidural anesthesia for cesarean delivery—immediate onset.
- Right dose in right space: After an unintentional dural puncture, the epidural catheter was inserted in a different space. During cesarean delivery, epidural local anesthetics enters sub-arachnoid space through the dural defect from concentration and pressure gradients—delayed onset.
- Wrong dose in right space: Excessive dose of local anesthetics in the epidural space, often in the situation of emergent cesarean delivery.

SYMPTOMS AND SIGNS—VARY AND PROGRESSIVE IN PRESENTATION

- Agitation to sudden loss of consciousness, coma, or seizures
- Muscle weakness, inability to speak to difficult of breathing to respiratory arrest
- Mild hypotension to cardiovascular collapse
- Bradycardia to cardiac arrest
- Paralysis and dysphasia
- Subdural block—may involve the cranial nerves; apnea and Horner's syndrome can occur

Of note, the physiologic changes in pregnancy lead to significant vasodilation; thus, the hypotension could be mild or absent. The onset of total spinal in the setting of an existing sympathectomy (e.g., after a labor epidural has been in place) may not cause further blood pressure derangement. Usually, inability to speak, agitation, mental status change, and arm/hand weakness are hallmarks of high neuraxial block.

PREVENTION AND TREATMENT (BOX 60-1)

- Continuous monitoring during labor and cesarean delivery.
- Maintain frequent verbal communication with the mother at all times.
- During labor epidural analgesia, the late onset of hypotension and significant muscle weakness in lower extremities must rule out the possibility of intrathecal catheter (Chapter 59, "Intrathecal Catheter").
- Administration of test dose and careful assessment of the patient's response.
- Aspiration of epidural catheter before every bolus.
- Incremental dosing of epidural catheter (5 mL each time)—every dose is a test dose.

BOX 60-1 • Management of High Spinal/Total Spinal

- Stop epidural infusion or bolus.
- Communicate with the team.
- Call for help.
- Airway: supplement oxygen to maintain oxygenation, tracheal intubation if indicated.
- Breathing: reverse Trendelenburg position to help breathing, maintaining patent airway.
- Circulation: left uterine displacement, a rapid intravenous fluid bolus, and administration of vasopressors to maintain hemodynamic stability.
- May consider delivering the baby.

References

1. D'Angelo R, Smiley RM, Riley ET, et al. Serious complications related to obstetric anesthesia. The serious complication repository project of the Society for Obstetric Anesthesia and Perinatology. *Anesthesiology*. 2014;120:1505-1512.
2. Hawkins JL, Chang J, Palmer SK, et al. Anesthesia-related maternal mortality in the United States: 1979-2002. *Obstet Gynecol*. 2011;117(1):69-74.
3. Davies JM, Posner KL, Lee LA, et al. Liability associated with obstetric anesthesia: a closed claims analysis. *Anesthesiology*. 2009;110:131-139.

61

Local Anesthetic Systemic Toxicity

Yunping Li, MD

BACKGROUND

- Incidence of local anesthetic systemic toxicity (LAST) after peripheral nerve blocks is higher than after epidural anesthesia.
- Ultrasound-guided peripheral nerve block is associated with lower incidence of LAST (Odds ratio 0.23).[1]
- Use of epinephrine in local anesthetics decreases its systemic absorption.
- In 1998, Dr. Guy Weinberg first observed that pretreatment or resuscitation with a lipid infusion shifts the dose-response curve to the right in a rat model of bupivacaine-induced asystole.[2]
- In 2006, the first case was reported of the successful use of a 20% lipid emulsion (intralipid) in a patient after LAST-induced prolong cardiac arrest.[3]
- Since then, lipid emulsion has been used successfully in lipophilic drug overdoses, such as tricyclic antidepressants, bupropion, verapamil, diltiazem, caffeine, and olanzapine.

RISK FACTORS

- Unrecognized intravascular epidural catheter
- Extremes of age
- Nerve block site
- Patient-related factors: cardiac, renal, and hepatic diseases
- Multiple procedures: such as labor analgesia to cesarean section, or regional block after cesarean section
- Multiple routes of administration: local infiltration, irrigation, neuraxial, nerve blocks, and lidocaine patch
- Repeated use of local anesthetics for infiltration

MECHANISM OF LIPID EMULSION (FIG. 61-1)[4]

- Lipid sink
- Metabolic effect: increases fatty acid uptake by mitochondria
- Membrane effect: stabilizes the membranes
- Cytoprotection: via activation of Protein kinase B (PKB), also known as Akt pathway

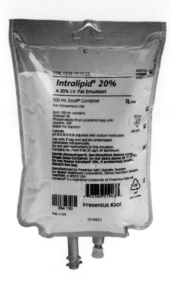

FIGURE 61-1 • Lipid emulsion: Intralipid.

DIAGNOSIS

The signs, symptoms, and timing of LAST are unpredictable and can be subtle. Wide range of symptoms include:

- Mental status change including coma and convulsions.
- Cardiovascular instability to cardiac arrest.
- **Be vigilant.** Early diagnosis is the key for successful resuscitation.

TREATMENT

- The LAST Checklist from the American Society of Regional Anesthesia and Pain Medicine (ASRA) summarizes the workflow of resuscitation of LAST and the use of lipid emulsion (Fig. 61-2).[5]
- Data are inconsistent regarding whether lipid emulsion is effective to resuscitate the patients with LAST due to lidocaine overdose. The lipid administration proved to be safe; the author would recommend using lipid emulsion to treat lidocaine-induced LAST.
- **Important note for resuscitation:** Use smaller than normal dose of epinephrine in the Advanced Cardiovascular Life Support (ACLS). Avoid beta blockers, calcium channel blockers, and vasopressin.

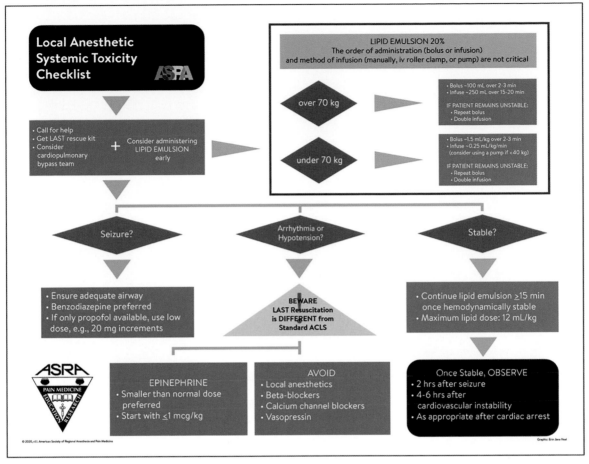

FIGURE 61-2 • ASRA-copyrighted LAST checklist and resuscitation workflow. (Reproduced with permission from American Society of Regional Anesthesia and Pain Medicine, ©2020.)

References

1. Barrington MJ, Kluger R. Ultrasound guidance reduces the risk of local anesthetic systemic toxicity following peripheral nerve blockade. *Reg Anesth Pain Med*. 2013;38:289-299.

2. Weinberg GL, VadeBoncouer T, Ramaraju GA, et al. Pretreatment or resuscitation with a lipid infusion shifts the dose-response to bupivacaine-induced asystole in rats. *Anesthesiology*. 1998;88(4):1071-1075.

3. Rosenblatt MA, Abel M, Fischer GW, et al. Successful use of a 20% lipid emulsion to resuscitate a patient after a presumed bupivacaine-related cardiac arrest. *Anesthesiology*. 2006;105(1):217-218.

4. Weinberg GL. Lipid emulsion infusion. *Anesthesiology*. 2012;117(1):180-187.

5. Neal JM, Neal EJ, Weinberg GL. American Society of Regional Anesthesia and Pain Medicine local anesthetic systemic toxicity checklist: 2020 version. *Reg Anesth Pain Med*. 2021;46:81-82.

62

Peripartum Neurological Complications

Maria C. Borrelli, DO
Philip E. Hess, MD

Most nerve injury after childbirth can be attributed to delivery of the neonate. These are referred to as *intrinsic obstetric palsies*, and are often due to stretching or compression of the lumbosacral plexus and lower extremity peripheral nerves. Fortunately, obstetric palsies are usually transient with expected full recovery. Rarely, potentially catastrophic neurological complications occur after neuraxial procedures. Prompt recognition and treatment are essential to avoid permanent injury.[1-3] Diagnosis and differential diagnosis of peripartum neurological injury are summarized in Fig. 62-1.

MILD COMPLICATIONS—MUSCULAR STRAIN

Myofascial pain syndrome: may occur in any region (common in neck, shoulders, lower extremities):

- Muscle hypertonicity/edema with marked tenderness at specific anatomic points
- Cervical myofascial pain, base of occiput, and neck pain without positional changes
- Management: Acetaminophen/Nonsteroidal anti-inflammatory drugs (NSAIDs), ice/heat, physical therapy (PT) consult

MODERATE COMPLICATIONS—PERIPHERAL NERVE INJURIES (TABLE 62-1)

- Associated with prolonged first or second stage of labor, difficult instrumental delivery, nulliparity, extremes of stature, and prolonged use of the lithotomy position
- Unilateral, with weakness/paralysis in single muscle or group of muscles
- Unilateral sensory deficits in nerve distribution
- May be bilateral, especially with plexus injuries
- Management: Conservative, consult PT with presence of muscle weakness

CATASTROPHIC COMPLICATIONS—CENTRAL LESIONS (FIG. 62-2)

Neurologic sequela of dural puncture (see Chapter 64, "Postdural Puncture Headache")

- Isolated cranial nerve palsies (cranial nerves VI and VIII most vulnerable), diplopia and/or tinnitus
  - Management: Epidural blood patch, emergent imaging if severe

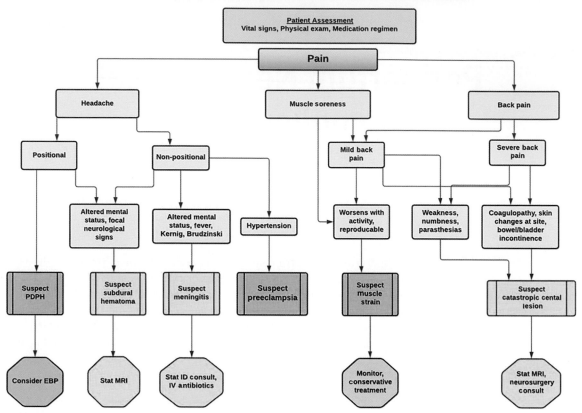

FIGURE 62-1 • Diagnosis of peripartum neurological injury. EBP, epidural blood patch; IV, intravenous; PDPH, postdural puncture headache; Stat MRI, emergent magnetic resonance imaging.

TABLE 62-1 • Characteristics of Peripheral Nerve Injury		
Nerve Palsy	**Symptoms**	**Possible Etiologies**
Lumbar plexus	Knee extension weakness, anterior thigh sensory deficit, can have saphenous nerve deficit, may be associated with hip flexion weakness and hydronephrosis	Cephalopelvic disproportion, prolonged labor, and difficult vaginal delivery
Sacral plexus	Sciatic distribution sensory deficit and weakness, foot drop	Compression of the plexus between the bony pelvis and fetal presenting part
Obturator	Weakness of hip adduction/internal rotation, sensory disturbance over medial thigh	Compression of the nerve between pelvis and fetal head, forceps delivery
Femoral	Weakness of hip flexion, patellar reflex is diminished/absent; sensory deficit of anterior thigh and medial calf	Stretch intrapelvic portion in lithotomy position or compress the nerve under the inguinal ligament or in the posterior iliopsoas region
Lateral femoral cutaneous (meralgia paresthetica)	Numbness, tingling, or burning sensation of the anterolateral aspect of the thigh	Entrapment of the nerve under the inguinal ligament by gravid uterus, retractors, obesity, or prolonged lithotomy position

TABLE 62-1 • Characteristics of Peripheral Nerve Injury		
Nerve Palsy	**Symptoms**	**Possible Etiologies**
Sciatic	Weakness and decreased sensation below the knee with sparing of the medial leg	Compression of nerve in buttock (piriformis) or posterior internal pelvis, stretch injury due to lithotomy position, prolonged sitting on a misplaced wedge
Peroneal (fibular)	Footdrop/weak ankle eversion, sensory deficit on the anterolateral calf and dorsum of the foot	Excessive knee flexion, compression of the lateral side of the knee, prolonged use of the lithotomy position (stirrup injury)

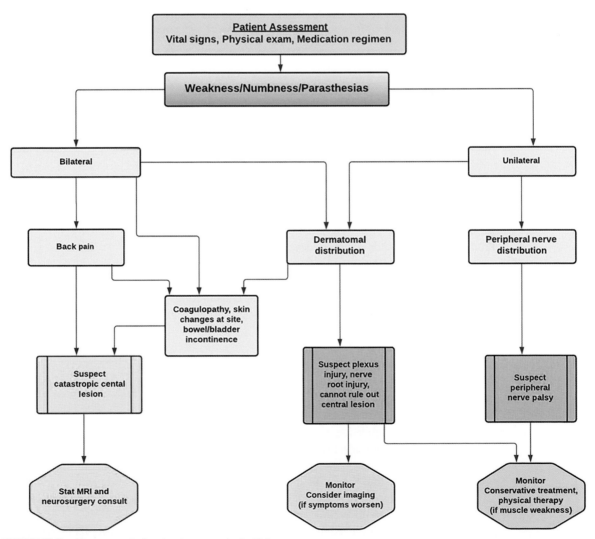

FIGURE 62-2 • Management of peripartum neurological injury.

- Subdural hematoma (rupture of bridge meningeal veins)
  - Persistent headache, focal neurologic signs present in majority of cases
  - Severe symptoms: Altered mental status, seizures, focal neurologic findings
  - Management: Emergent imaging, neurosurgery consultation
- Cortical vein and venous sinus thrombosis: Can be associated with postdural puncture headache

Infectious etiologies

- Epidural abscess
  - Risk factors: Prolonged catheterization, poor aseptic technique, multiple attempts at insertion, traumatic insertion, no bacterial filter, immunocompromised patients
  - Likely to present 3 to 5 days after the procedure
  - Severe backache ($+/-$ local tenderness), fever, radicular pain/numbness at lower extremities, catheter entry point inflamed $+/-$ fluid leak/purulence
  - Labs: Leukocytosis, increased c-reactive protein
  - Management: Emergent imaging, antibiotics, neurosurgery consultation
- Meningitis
  - Risk factors: Dural puncture, labor, no face mask during placement, manual removal of the placenta, vaginal infection
  - 12 hours to 2 days postpartum
  - Fever, headache, photophobia, nausea, vomiting, neck stiffness, confusion, drowsiness, Kernig's sign (inability to straighten the knee when the hip is flexed)
  - Management: Infectious disease consult, antibiotics, supportive care

Vascular etiologies

- Subdural hematoma: See above
- Epidural hematoma: Difficult/traumatic epidural needle/catheter placement, coagulopathy/anticoagulation, spinal deformity, spinal tumor
  - From 24 to 48 hours for symptom development
  - Symptoms: Severe back pain, significant delay in sensory and motor recovery $+/-$ deterioration of lower extremity or bladder function
  - Management: Emergent imaging, neurosurgery consultation

Chemical etiologies

- Transient neurologic symptoms
  - Risk factors: Intrathecal lidocaine, lithotomy
  - Presentation: 1 to 10 days with pain in back, buttocks, thighs without sensory/motor dysfunction, typically lasts 2 to 3 days, self-limiting
  - Management: Supportive
- Arachnoiditis: Rare complication caused by inflammation of arachnoid[4]
  - Risk factors: Inadvertent injection of skin antiseptic solution into the epidural space, accidental intrathecal injection of potentially neurotoxic local anesthetic, unintentional injection/spread of blood into the dural/subdural space during epidural blood patch
  - Varies in symptom onset, may present with severe pain during procedure with progressive severe back pain and neurological symptoms (over days to weeks)
  - Management: Supportive, need to exclude other catastrophic central lesions via imaging (magnetic resonance imaging is gold standard)

Direct trauma

- Direct trauma to the spinal cord, conus medullaris, and nerve roots can be a result of spinal or epidural needle injury

References

1. Sviggum H, Reynolds F. Neurologic complications of pregnancy and neuraxial anesthesia. In: *Chestnut's Obstetric Anesthesia: Principles and Practice*. 6th ed. Philadelphia, PA: Elsevier; 2020:752-776.
2. Wong CA. Nerve injuries after neuraxial anaesthesia and their medicolegal implications. *Best Pract Res Clin Obstet Gynaecol*. 2010;24:367-381.
3. Loo CC, Dahlgren G, Irestedt L. Neurological complications in obstetric regional anaesthesia. *Int J Obstet Anesth*. 2000; 9:99-124.
4. Killeen T, Kamat A, Walsh D, et al. Severe adhesive arachnoiditis resulting in progressive paraplegia following obstetric spinal anaesthesia: a case report and review. *Anaesthesia*. 2012;67:1386.

63

Aspiration

Anna Moldysz, MD

BACKGROUND

Aspiration of gastric contents can cause a chemical pneumonitis characterized by tachypnea, hypoxia, and fever, first described by Mendelson in 1946.[1] The incidence of mortality from aspiration during anesthesia for labor and delivery has declined over the recent decades. Data from *Mothers and Babies—Reducing Risk through Audits and Confidential Enquiries across the UK* (MBRRACE-UK), which is the most comprehensive database on maternal mortality, suggests aspiration has **not** been a contributing factor to maternal mortality since 2009.[2] The Serious Complication Repository Project in the United States evaluated 257,000 deliveries at 30 institutions between 2004 and 2009, found **no** reported cases of aspiration.[3] This decline is likely due to:

- The greater use of neuraxial techniques for cesarean delivery
- The frequent use of chemical prophylaxis
- Rapid sequence intubation in the event of a general anesthetic
- Better anesthesia training
- Adherence to NPO (nothing by mouth) guidelines[4]

The true incidences of aspiration and aspiration pneumonitis are difficult to determine because of inconsistent criteria for diagnosis and lack of comprehensive data. However, it is known that morbidity varies according to ASA status of the patient, the type and volume of aspirate, the therapy administered, and criteria for diagnosis. This chapter will primarily focus on how to identify parturients at risk for aspiration and administer prophylaxis as indicated to reduce the risk of complications.

RISK FACTORS FOR ASPIRATION[5]

- Inadequate fasting time
- Emergency surgery
- General anesthesia, especially with difficult intubation
- Gastrointestinal obstruction
- Previous gastrointestinal surgery
- Delayed gastric emptying (i.e., diabetes, active labor, opioids)
- Recent trauma
- Increased intracranial pressure
- Morbid obesity
- Use of nitrous during labor
- Cognitive neurological impairment

GASTRIC ULTRASOUND

- Gastric ultrasound has been studied, but not yet fully validated for assessment of aspiration risk in obstetrics.
- There may be a role for gastric ultrasound in cases of urgent cesarean delivery for women who have not met fasting guidelines.
- If a nonfasted parturient has a full stomach on ultrasound, delay surgery if possible, avoid general anesthesia if possible, and consider additional promotility agents.

PROPHYLAXIS

- If possible, adhere to NPO guidelines (see Chapter 36, "NPO Guidelines").
- Use neuraxial anesthesia whenever possible, and advocate early labor epidural for high-risk parturients.
- For induction of general anesthesia, use rapid sequence induction and tracheal intubation.
- Under general anesthesia, empty stomach using orogastric tube prior to extubation and extubate awake after return of airway reflexes—risk of aspiration at extubation is equal to that of induction (Chapter 48, "General Anesthesia for Cesarean Delivery").
- "Consider the timely administration of nonparticulate antacids, H2-receptor antagonists, and/or metoclopramide for aspiration prophylaxis"—ASA Practice Guidelines for Obstetric Anesthesia[6,7] (see Table 63-1).

TABLE 63-1 • Chemical Prophylaxis Against Aspiration Pneumonitis

Agent	Mechanism	Dose	Timing	Considerations
Nonparticulate Antacids Sodium bicarbonate Sodium citrate	Reduces acidity of gastric contents	30 mL sodium citrate (Bicitra)	Administer within 20 minutes of induction of GA	Duration of action depends on rate of gastric emptying
Histamine-2 Receptor Antagonists Famotidine Ranitidine	Block H2 receptors on oxyntic cell to decrease gastric acid production	Famotidine: 20-40 mg PO or IV Ranitidine: 50-100 mg IV or 150 mg PO	Onset: 30 minutes (IV) Maximum effect: 60-90 minutes	Long duration of action (>8 hours), will last through emergence if GA
Proton Pump Inhibitors Omeprazole Lansoprazole	Inhibit hydrogen ion pump on gastric surface of oxyntic cell	Omeprazole: 20-40 mg PO Lansoprazole: 15-30 mg PO	Onset: 30 minutes	Long duration of action, low toxicity Less effective than ranitidine in increasing pH and decreasing gastric volume[7]
Metoclopramide	Peripheral cholinergic agonist, central dopamine receptor antagonist Increases lower esophageal sphincter tone and increases gastric peristalsis	10 mg IV	Onset: 15 minutes	Prior administration of opioid or atropine antagonizes the effect Can cause extrapyramidal symptoms

GA, general anesthesia; PO, nothing by mouth.

References

1. Mendelson CL. The aspiration of stomach contents into the lungs during obstetric anesthesia. *Am. J Obstet Gynec.* 1946;52:191-205.

2. Knight M, Bunch K, Tuffnell D, et al. (eds) on behalf of MBRRACE-UK. *Saving lives, improving mothers' care - lessons learned to inform maternity care from the UK and Ireland Confidential Enquiries into Maternal Deaths and Morbidity 2017-19.* Oxford: National Perinatal Epidemiology Unit, University of Oxford; 2021.

3. D'Angelo R, Smiley RM, Riley ET, Segal S. Serious complications related to obstetric anesthesia: the serious complication repository project of the Society for Obstetric Anesthesia and Perinatology. *Anesthesiology.* 2014;120(6): 1505-1512.

4. Farber M. Aspiration: risk, prophylaxis, and treatment. In: *Chestnut's Obstetric Anesthesia Principles and Practice.* 6th ed. Philadelphia, PA: Elsevier; 2020:671-687.

5. Robinson M, Davidson A. Aspiration under anaesthesia: risk assessment and decision-making. *Continuing Education in Anaesthesia, Critical Care & Pain.* 2014;14(4):171-175.

6. Practice Guidelines for Obstetric Anesthesia: An Updated Report by the American Society of Anesthesiologists Task Force on Obstetric Anesthesia and the Society for Obstetric Anesthesia and Perinatology. *Anesthesiology.* 2016;124(2):270-300.

7. Clark K, Lam LT, Gibson S, Currow D. The effect of ranitidine versus proton pump inhibitors on gastric secretions: a meta-analysis of randomised control trials. *Anaesthesia.* 2009;64(6):652-657.

64

Postdural Puncture Headache

Vimal K. Akhouri, MD
Yunping Li, MD

BACKGROUND

The incidence of postdural puncture headache (PDPH) varies widely, depending on patient population, the experience level of care providers, and the size and type of the needle. The Society for Obstetric Anesthesia and Perinatology Center of Excellence sets the benchmark rate of unintentional dural puncture (UDP) at $\leq 2\%$.

The mechanism of PDPH after unintentional dural puncture (UDP) derives from leakage of cerebrospinal fluid (CSF), resulting in low CSF pressure. In the upright position, low CSF pressure causes vascular dilation and the loss of cushioning effect leads to stretching intracranial vasculature and cranial nerves. The most commonly affected cranial nerves are the abducens nerve (VI) and vestibulocochlear nerve (VIII); both nerves are prone to stretch and compression due to their long path at the cranial base.

Prompt treatment of PDPH can greatly improve maternal recovery after delivery and enhance the ability to take care of newborn babies. Although untreated PDPH can resolve within 2 weeks, severe adverse outcomes, such as subdural hematoma, can occur. Fortunately, these have an extremely low incidence.[1] Recent evidence shows PDPH may be associated with long-term headache, backache, and depression.[2]

RISK FACTORS OF PDPH

- Female gender
- Pregnancy
- Younger age
- Low body mass index (BMI): higher incidence of UDP due to much shorter distance from the skin to epidural space; higher incidence of PDPH after UDP due to greater pressure gradient between lumbar CSF pressure and epidural pressure compared to high BMI patients
- Needle size: the incidence of PDPH can be as high as 81% to 88% after UDP with 17G epidural needle in pregnant women[3]
- Shape and orientation of the needle tip

DIAGNOSIS OF PDPH

- Positional headache that occurs within 5 days after a dural puncture. The positional nature is no longer required for diagnosis due to ~10% atypical headache.[4]

- Positional neck pain/stiffness, with or without headache, is also diagnostic.
- PDPH can be accompanied by photophobia, diplopia, nausea, vomiting, and subjective hearing symptoms.
- Headache that is not better accounted for by other causes in the postpartum period, including stress/tension headache, caffeine withdrawal, sleep deprivation, migraine headache, preeclampsia, subarachnoid hemorrhage, and cortical vein thrombosis.

NEUROLOGIC COMPLICATIONS ASSOCIATED WITH PDPH[5]

UDP and PDPH increase the risks of the following neurologic complications:

- Cerebral venous thrombosis (odds ratios [OR] 19)
- Subdural hematoma (OR 19)
- Bacterial meningitis (OR 39.7)
- Persistent chronic headache
- Possible permanent diplopia or hearing change

TREATMENT OF POSTDURAL PUNCTURE HEADACHE (FIG. 64-1)

The goals to actively treat PDPH:

- Alleviate the symptoms and allow mothers to take care of their newborns.
- Prevent neurological complications, such as subdural hematoma, hearing change, and diplopia.

Epidural blood patch (EBP) is considered the definitive management for PDPH. Sphenopalatine ganglion block has been described for symptomatic alleviation, although the benefits are often short-lived.[6,7] Cosyntropin (1 mg IV over 20 minutes) has also been described for prevention of PDPH after UDP, but has limited data.[6]

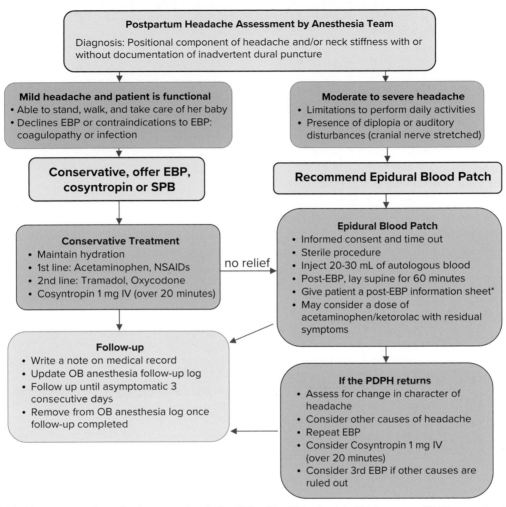

FIGURE 64-1 • Management of postdural puncture headache. EBP, epidural blood patch; IV, intravenous; NSAIDs, nonsteroidal anti-inflammatory drugs; SPB, sphenopalatine.

*See Chapter 65, "Patient Information: Unintentional Dural Puncture."

Patients with PDPH should be followed up daily till full recovery. Post-EBP instructions are included in Box 64-1.

BOX 64-1 • Post-EBP Instructions

- No heavy lifting, bending, or straining for the first 48 hours after epidural blood patch.
- Take ibuprofen (Advil) and acetaminophen (Tylenol), as needed for back discomfort. Do not take more than 600 mg of ibuprofen every 6 hours or more than 1000 mg of acetaminophen every 8 hours.
- You may shower.
- If you have symptoms of fever, chills, worsening headache, and/or severe back pain, please call your obstetrician's office immediately.
- Expect a call from an Obstetric Anesthesiologist the next day to follow-up.
- If you have further questions/concerns about blood patch, please feel free to call Labor and Delivery Unit and ask for an Obstetric Anesthesiologist. The team is here 24 hours a day and are happy to address your questions/concerns as soon as possible.

References

1. Moore AR, Wieczorek PM, Carvalho JCA. Association between post-dural puncture headache after neuraxial anesthesia in childbirth and intracranial subdural hematoma. *JAMA Neurol*. 2020;77(1):65-72.
2. Mims SC, Tan HS, Sun K, et al. Long-term morbidities following unintentional dural puncture in obstetric patients: a systematic review and meta-analysis. *J Clin Anesth*. 2022;79:110787.
3. Bateman BT, Cole N, Sun-Edelstein C, et al. Post dural puncture headache. UpToDate. Accessed April 2022.
4. The International Headache Society. The third edition of the international classification of headache disorders (ICHD-3) 7.2.1. Post-lumbar puncture headache. Accessed April 2022.
5. Guglielminotti J, Landau R, Li G. Major neurologic complications associated with postdural puncture headache in obstetrics: a retrospective cohort study. *Anesth Analg*. 2019;129:1328-1336.
6. Russell R, Laxton C, Lucas DN, et al. Treatment of obstetric post-dural puncture headache. Part 1: conservative and pharmacological management. *Int J Obstet Anesth*. 2019;38:93-103.
7. Russell R, Laxton C, Lucas DN, et al. Treatment of obstetric post-dural puncture headache. Part 2: epidural blood patch. *Int J Obstet Anesth*. 2019;38:104-118.

65

Patient Information: Unintentional Dural Puncture

Philip E. Hess, MD

During the placement of your epidural, a layer around the spinal fluid, called the *dura*, was punctured with a needle unintentionally. The puncture of the dura happens on occasion during epidural placement. The hole allows spinal fluid to slowly drain.

You are at risk of developing a "spinal" headache.

A spinal headache usually starts 1 to 3 days after the puncture of the dura and can range from mild to severe. The headache is usually felt in the front or back of the head or may even cause a muscle cramping between your shoulder blades or your neck. It gets worse when you stand or sit. It improves or goes away when you lie down.

Other symptoms may include nausea and vomiting, ringing in your ears, fullness/blocked feeling in your ears, sensitivity to light, and double vision.

Your anesthesiology team can discuss treatment options with you.

The team will follow up with you closely. If you develop a headache, please call:

- Obstetric Anesthesia Office
- Labor and Delivery
- Department of Anesthesia

Ask for the obstetric anesthesiologist. You may also call your obstetrician, who can get in touch with the team.

Things you should know:

- These headaches typically go away without treatment; however, it can take days to a couple of weeks.
- The most effective treatment is an epidural blood patch, which your anesthesiologist can explain in detail.
- Drink enough water to avoid being dehydrated. Eat and sleep to the best of your ability as you would normally.
- Do not stand for prolonged periods of time, even if the headache is mild.
- If the headache is severe or you think you need treatment, please contact obstetric anesthesiologist.
- You can use acetaminophen (Tylenol) or ibuprofen (Advil) for pain control, if you do not have any other contraindications to these medications. Do not take more than 600 mg of ibuprofen every 6 hours or more than 1000 mg of acetaminophen every 8 hours.
- You may also try caffeine.

Index